FACING DEATH

Finding Dignity, Hope and Healing at the End

Jim deMaine

TABLE OF CONTENTS

To Lourdes, my loving wife and best friend

"Death is no more than passing from one room into another. But there's a difference for me, you know. Because in the other room, I shall be able to see."

—Helen Keller

AUTHOR'S NOTE

This book is non-fiction. In some cases, names and identifying features have been changed in order to respect privacy. Portions of the book have been published on my blog www.endoflifeblog.com between 2009 and 2020.

FOREWORD

Why is death so hard? Or perhaps it's just dying that's really hard. After all, everyone knows that death is inevitable. Every day we live, we're one day closer to dying, of course. But that's not the way most people think. Maybe the hard part is that death is frightening, and unless we're actively facing it—either with our own illness or through that of a loved one—we just don't want to confront it.

But death is inevitable. Dying is literally part of living. Fortunately, we now have this book, *Facing Death: Finding Dignity, Hope and Healing at the End*. It's a down to earth and invaluable resource for learning more about death. It's also, perhaps counter-intuitively, a delight to read. Jim deMaine is a seasoned internist who spent his career in pulmonary and critical care medicine. For thirty-eight years he cared for very sick and terminally ill patients. Those experiences inform his insights, and they are presented with stories about the good and not-so-good journeys of Jim's patients, family and friends through death and dying. Jim also describes his personal journey as an idealistic, young physician who became today's revered internist. I've learned much from this wise teller of true stories, and I hope it will be read by clinicians of every ilk in training and in practice. But its most immediate value will be to those confronting their own imminent passing or that of a loved one. The notion of a good death is highly individual. Each one of us will have a unique view of how it should look and feel.

For example, my father-in-law, who founded a volunteer clinic devoted to serving low-income patients in Newark, New Jersey, observed about growing old: "You get to be my age and you understand that aging is gradual dying." I discuss this point of view in my own book, Enlightened Aging, and they are reiterated through the words of poet Wallace Stevens who wrote, "Death is the mother of beauty." Stevens is pointing out the ways we see beauty in those things that are limited, fleeting. One of the great lessons of aging is the realization that life gets better—more beautiful—when we accept that our time may be short.

In my own medical practice, I often heard people say that a "good death" would be going to sleep and just not waking up. Yet, when a younger or middle-aged person dies this way, unexpectedly, survivors experience great grief, disabling shock, and often clinical depression. For those people who have an expected death, preceded by a recognizable process of decline, spouses and other loved ones don't suffer the same emotional extremes. Is that a "good death"?

In 1969, Elizabeth Kubler-Ross famously moved awareness of death into everyday medical training with her best-selling book, On Death and Dying. Her work made an indelible impression on me as a medical student—especially her observation that what people most fear about death is being abandoned at the end. This has profound resonance for us today, in the wake of Covid-19. But it bears remembering for all of us, at any time: there is great value for doctors, patients, and families to think about and express our wishes around death and how we will die.

With modern medicine, ever-larger numbers of people are living deep into old age with progressive illnesses that in many instances will lead to death. Meaning that the "good death" idea of someday just not waking up is increasingly unusual. So what, then, is good death?

A report from the National Academy of Science's Institute of Medicine, "Dying in America: Improving Quality and Honoring Individual Preferences Near the End of Life," concludes that the U.S. health care system is poorly designed to meet the needs of patients and their families. Although there has been great improvement in establishing programs for palliative and hospice care, the report calls for radical reforms in education on promoting more meaningful discussions between patients and clinicians around end-of-life planning. As a society, we tend to be "at war with death," the report says, which isn't surprising since that attitude characterizes modern health care. Even though we know it's a war we will never win.

A better approach would be to consider the type of care we will want late in life, when we realize our time may be short. At that point, we begin to understand that life does get better with a shift in perspective. We begin to consider our preferences for care, especially in the case of painful, progressive, or terminal illness.

An unusually informative paper called "Defining a good death" surveyed thousands of dying people and their family members and concluded that among many features of "successful dying," the ones most highly regarded were honoring patient wishes, being free of pain, and promoting emotional wellbeing. This work, published in 2016, called for more research and public conversation because there are tremendous differences of opinion on this topic. Jim deMaine's book is a valuable contribution to that effort.

There is no single best way to die. We are all individuals with different lives and perspectives. But I think most of us can agree that people experience this phase of life more peacefully when they have given some thought and made provisions for their wishes beforehand. Reading *Facing Death: Finding Dignity, hope and Healing at the End* will give readers a window onto the experiences of many families, providing examples for how you might want things to go—or not go.

In America, we are masters of individualism. We have built an entire national ethos around living life on our own terms. Why wouldn't we extend that approach to the moment of ultimate culmination, our own deaths? In that way, we might best understand Wallace Stevens' realization that death really can be a way toward seeing the beauty and great gift of life.

Eric Larson
Seattle, 2020

INTRODUCTION

For thirty-eight years I cared for very sick, terminally ill patients. Their stories—their deaths and suffering—have become part of me. I have collected and treasured the many kind notes that patients and families have sent me, at times crediting me with powers I do not deserve. As I ministered to patients, their loved ones and caregivers, I was part doctor, part teacher, and part spiritual advisor. In a care conference in the ICU, I would often tell a story to help a family understand the crisis their loved one was enduring. I tend to think in stories and found that, through them, families could more easily grasp whatever lesson I was trying to impart. They, like most of us, had not talked much about death and were unprepared for it. But when death lands on our doorstep, do we lock the door or welcome it in? Dying is different for each of us as we enter the unknowable on our own unique path.

Sometimes we negotiate. Larry surprised me during a visit to my pulmonary clinic. "Doc, I want to take you out to lunch. There's something I want to discuss with you."

I was a little nervous about the invitation. Larry was a favorite patient of mine, coming across as a bit crusty but a straight shooter. I'd grown to know him well and we often chatted about his former career in sales. I was a bit concerned that he might try to sell me something—and in a way, he did.

We arranged to meet at a restaurant near the hospital, and after some pleasantries, Larry let me know that he wanted to talk about dying.

"Look, I've lived a long time and what I'm doing now isn't really living," he said. "These flare-ups are torture. I feel like a fish out of water and I don't want to die that way. My biggest fear is suffocating to death. Doc, I want you to help me at the end."

Larry was suffering from severe COPD, and his condition was getting worse. He had a piercing gaze that twinkled when he cracked one of his frequent jokes, and he always appeared well groomed. But he breathed noisily and had a dusky color, even with the oxygen flowing through his nasal prongs. Larry was not joking now. He'd just been discharged from the hospital after another crisis, with severe wheezing, gasping and coughing due to infection. His waterfront home, where he lived alone at age seventy-seven, had become a prison to him.

"Doc, I can't handle the stairs, go crabbing, or even lean over to dig clams. This is the pits."

"How about hiring live-in help or moving to Seattle to be closer to your family and medical care?"

"No way," Larry said. "I don't want to move and bother my sons or have some stranger in my home!"

Larry's COPD was near end stage. He had the classic findings of distended neck veins and a barrel-shaped chest. His lungs were over-expanded, and his diaphragms were moving poorly. There was a trace of swelling in his legs. His blood showed elevated carbon dioxide, and he couldn't breathe well enough either to maintain oxygen or expel CO_2. Chronic respiratory failure due to longstanding tobacco use was his diagnosis. He had finally kicked the habit five years earlier, which helped some, but not enough. Looking at him, I could see the side effects of prescribed steroids—the "moon face," bruising of the arms, muscle wasting and weakness—all scourges of chronic use of prednisone.

We talked about ventilators to support his breathing and other kinds of ICU care. "No," he said. Larry was clear; he wanted to be in control. "Look Doc, all I want you to do is promise me that you'll help me at the end."

I continued to listen as he explained his feelings and fears. He didn't appear significantly depressed, but I needed to check. "Larry, do you feel sad or hopeless?"

He replied, "No, just mad as hell that I can't get better."

I felt that Larry had very natural "situational depression" from his illness and I suggested a low dose antidepressant, but he refused—perhaps because of the medication's unpleasant side effects, perhaps because he did not think he was particularly despondent.

So we discussed options for what would now be called aggressive palliative care. "Larry, look I'm not Dr. Kevorkian, but there are options. Other than the medications and oxygen you are using to help you breathe, the best drug at the end is morphine. This drug takes away the suffocating feeling, treats any pain, sedates you, and produces euphoria."

"Well, Doc, that's what I want."

"Ok, but there's a catch. Morphine would likely speed up your death by several hours—or even days. If your aim is to relieve suffering, drugs like morphine will work. But they can hasten death."

Larry was resolute. "Look, I just want to die comfortably," he said. "I know I'm dying so what's a few less hours or days?"

Later, when recounting our discussion to a few of my colleagues, I got a mixed response. One said, "There are situations you just can't jump into. This is too close to assisted suicide."

But another felt patients should have the right to ask for relief from suffering. "After all, since you can't cure him you are at least obligated to relieve his intolerable symptoms."

A religious scholar friend had a broad view. "Your patient is suffering, and you have tools to help him. I don't think it's wise to abandon him in his time of need. He'll be transitioning from this life to the next soon enough. Why extend his needless suffering?"

I tentatively agreed to comply with Larry's wishes whenever his next inevitable flare-up occurred. But I insisted that he try to get buy-in from his two sons, one an attorney and the other a veterinarian. A week later I conferred with Larry and his sons who agreed with their dad's plan. And then we waited.

Seattle gets dark very early during the Christmas season, and this is when my pulmonary practice always seemed busiest. Pneumonias were at a peak. New lung cancers were constantly showing up. The sad stories were relentless. Every day, my anger at tobacco companies flared hotter. But my spirits were buoyed by a significant skirmish we'd recently won. It was 1983, and smoking finally had been banned at my hospital. Prior to that, doctors puffed on cigarettes while making their rounds, and incredible as it sounds today, families smoked in patient rooms.

At dinner two days before Christmas, I got a phone call at home from the ER doctor. Larry had been admitted, and they were preparing to put him in the ICU. I said, "I'm not sure he wants to go there. Please hold him in the ER, and I'll come see him."

At his bedside shortly thereafter, I could see that Larry looked awful. "Remember what you promised," he rasped, his piercing eyes intent as ever.

I reviewed our plan aloud, and Larry nodded. Normally he would have gone to intensive care, but we would bypass that and admit him directly to a medical unit with a do-not-resuscitate (DNR) order.

I pulled the nurses aside and explained the situation. Fortunately, they were senior caregivers, models of caring and competence. They had seen too many cases of CPR used on terminal patients—a violent and jarring experience for all—and they were relieved to be free of that obligation. "Doctor, I'm glad you don't view death as a failure in this situation," one said. God bless nurses. They were looking after me!

The morphine drip was started with small supplements as needed. Larry's sons were there. Larry himself seemed peaceful, and on my drive home I said a silent prayer. I slept well that night. Larry passed from this world at 3:14 AM.

I offer this story as a way into discussing the ethics of offering palliative treatments that likely hasten death. Key to this question is intent.[1] In 1983, when I was caring for Larry, there were no clear guidelines so I had to rely on my own training, intuition, and personal comfort zone. And though various groups have published guidelines in recent years,[2] they are still not completely clear.

What we gave Larry is now called "palliative sedation," a term aimed at emphasizing the physician's intent to ease suffering, rather than intentionally cause a patient's death. This kind of sedation differs from assisted suicide precisely because of that one word, *intent*. This is called the double effect. The intent is to relieve pain even if a secondary effect is to hasten death. Some people deride this distinction as splitting hairs. But in 1997, the U.S. Supreme Court gave strong support for this principle in its deliberations about the constitutionality of medical aid in dying.[3] The thinking in bioethics continues to evolve on this topic.[4]

I was deeply touched by the letter of thanks from Larry's two sons that came a few weeks after his death. "Dad would love to shake your hand if he could," they wrote. "He died the way he wanted to. Thanks and God bless."

Larry's story is one of many that I share in this book. His dying went well, but all too often our wishes around end-of-life arrangements aren't clear. Worse, sometimes they are disregarded. What if I had not been available? Would my colleagues have done the same? What if Larry's sons had not agreed? What if Larry himself had not so bravely and directly helped to guide his own dying?

We only die once—hopefully. Modern medical technology can prolong death, maybe even reverse its tide temporarily. But when we're talking about a person's final breath, there is only one. Generally, dying isn't something we can practice, and it's not something we discuss much. Most people actively try to avoid any thought of it. But dying will happen. As noted by humorists at *The Onion*,[5] the world death rate is holding steady at 100%.

Today, we mostly understand death as something happening to others while we deal with the more immediate cares of our lives. But in eras past, death was a common companion, always lurking around the corner. It has touched the hearts of many writers: Kipling spoke to the horrors of war in *A Death Bed*; Walt Whitman expressed his grief over the death of President Lincoln in *O Captain! My Captain!*; and John Donne felt that "We wake eternally and death shall be no more" in *Death, Be Not Proud*. Indeed, disease and death often are central features in literature, opera, art, and religious thought. In the not too distant past, tuberculosis, a common cause of death, inspired great novels and operas—Thomas Mann's *The Magic Mountain* and Puccini's *La Boehme*, for example. Unfortunately, TB continues to take more than one million lives annually in developing nations.

Until the COVID-19 pandemic, heart disease and cancer were the leading causes of death in developed countries. But in early 2020, the world was suddenly turned upside down. No one, of any age, was immune to a new strain of coronavirus that originated in China. It engendered a worldwide panic unknown since the influenza epidemic of 1918, and quickly became a leading cause of death in America. The COVID-19 pandemic has forced many to confront death and its painful losses more suddenly than they had anticipated, particularly among Black and Latinx communities. However, most of us won't die from the ravages of COVID-19. We are much more likely to die of a chronic illness in our old age.

Aging itself is loss. We experience it as a prelude to death. Our muscles weaken along with our bones, vision and hearing. We become forgetful. We lose balance, and we worry. We see friends pass away, attend memorials, and begin to wonder about our own. Medical appointments fill our schedules. Aging is supposed to bring wisdom. But in the age of social media—where attention spans are shorter and the pace of life exponentially faster—it feels more difficult than ever to cope with death creeping closer to our front door.

Shakespeare wrote eloquently about aging and loss in his 73rd sonnet.

> *That time of year thou mayst in me behold*
> *When yellow leaves, or none, or few, do hang*
> *Upon those boughs which shake against the cold,*
> *Bare ruin'd choirs, where late the sweet birds sang.*
> *In me thou seest the twilight of such day*

As after sunset fadeth in the west,
Which by and by black night doth take away,
Death's second self, that seals up all in rest.
In me thou see'st the glowing of such fire
That on the ashes of his youth doth lie,
As the death-bed whereon it must expire
Consumed with that which it was nourish'd by.
  This thou perceivest, which makes thy love more strong,
  To love that well which thou must leave ere long.

In grade school, as a class assignment, I chose this sonnet to memorize, but didn't understand the metaphors until much later. *"To love that well which thou must leave ere long."* This is the basis of pre-grief that affects us often as we face aspects of our aging, and often failing bodies.

Must approaching old age invariably be depressing? Not at all. Recent studies of aging and loss offer hope for a better quality of life, even as we age. Eric Larson's book, *Enlightened Aging: Building Resilience for a Long, Active Life,* offers ways to enhance wellbeing as we age. Among them: proactively managing our health; focusing on relationships and ways to be useful; and building up our personal reservoirs of mental, physical, and social health.

But can we expand beyond Larson's research on enlightened aging? What more can we say about death itself? Sherwin B. Nuland's *How We Die: Reflections on Life's Final Chapter* addresses dying from his vantage point as a surgeon and historian. Death may be dignified, he writes, but it often involves some degree of physical and emotional suffering. "The art of dying is the art of living," he says. "The honesty and grace of the years of life that are ending is the real measure of how we die."[6]

In this book I present my own stories, lessons learned from patients like Larry and many others who taught me about dying. My medical career began in an era when little could be done for two of our greatest killers—heart disease and cancer. There were no ventilators. I often saw patients die without the benefit of hospice care. ICUs and CCUs had not yet evolved. But with amazing rapidity, medical science has brought us life-saving advances such as hemodialysis and organ transplants. This progress is both marvelous and problematic, as technology continually outpaces our ability to thoughtfully and ethically bring it to the bedside. When should life-prolonging advances be used? How do we decide to whom to allocate these tools when resources are scarce or prohibitively expensive?

My stories are about hopes and fears common to us all. They are about the ethical dilemmas I've encountered and moments that have humbled me. They address advance care planning, medical aid-in-dying, conflicts, medical mistakes, modern hospice, and palliative care. They can be read in the order presented or topically, as relevant to each person's immediate questions and concerns. In the last section, I share my thoughts about resilience and leaving a legacy to our loved ones.

As I wrote about these patients and my experiences with them, memories surged to the surface of my thoughts, often bringing up deeply rooted feelings of sadness and joy, even fear. Did I do the right thing? Was I losing empathy? I hope as you read these stories that they encourage you to talk to your loved ones about your own hopes and fears. My greatest wish is to generate some much needed conversation about the inevitable and the choices we must consider. There is no easy way to put it: to ensure that our autonomy is respected, each of us must choose our path at the end.

MY STORY

*W**hy did I become a doctor? In retrospect, I never really seriously considered another profession. At times I have not found it easy to be around death so much. I didn't choose a "happy specialty" like obstetrics or ophthalmology or a low stress specialty like dermatology. A winding path led me to intensive care, a specialty that didn't even exist when I started out. I could have been a story with many different endings.*

BECOMING A DOCTOR

I was seventeen years old when I witnessed my first death as an orderly at Akron General Hospital during the summer. I had worked in Mr. Albrecht's room off and on for about a week. He was being treated for pneumonia with a new sulfa antibiotic. One day I walked in to change his bed and found him unconscious. Panicked, I ran to the nurses' station, and a page went out to the house doctor to come stat.

The intern arrived and examined him. "Well, there's no heartbeat. He's gone. I think it was his liver." That was that in 1955. No CPR in those days. My reaction was confusion. What had happened? Could anything have been done? I think it was then that I decided I wanted to learn more. How do we die? What happens to the dying person? I was wheeling the gurney down to the morgue later as I pondered these questions. I wasn't delving into the mystery of an afterlife. It was simply, how can we be here one moment and gone the next?

At the time, I'd avoided thinking much about what I would do with my life, and I certainly did not envision becoming a doctor like my father. His life as a general practitioner seemed arduous, his path to that point—college, medical school, and specialty training—just impossible. At home, the phone would ring at all hours. I'd hear Dad's car leaving at midnight to check on a woman in labor. I didn't think I'd ever want to work that hard. But other things did leave an impression. I'd see patients come by the house with some eggs or corn when behind on their bills. Following Dad around, I'd absorb the pungent smell of hospital ether and the strange odor of antiseptics in his office. But I put off thinking about actually becoming a doctor. Procrastination was my nature. Also, I didn't yet believe that I had what it took to follow in my father's footsteps.

As an orderly, I did a little of everything at the direction of Miss Dedinato, very definitely an I'm-in-charge kind of nurse. At her command, I transported patients, made beds, served dinner trays, and gave bed baths. I shaved a patient's head before he was taken for brain surgery and learned later that he remained in a coma. Miss D., as we called her, was kind but patrolled her ward like a drill sergeant to ensure that it ran smoothly. This was my first realization of the importance of nurses. They are the absolute backbone of patient care.

The hospital's patients were often talkative, sometimes telling me about their health and personal issues. But they'd clam up when the doctor came in, rushing through his charts and questions. (The doctors were almost always men in those days.) At times, I felt the patients were confiding in me more than in their doctor, a lesson that stuck with me.

My mom had always encouraged me to read, and one of the books that affected me most was Morton Thompson's *The Cry and the Covenant*. Women were dying from infections at childbirth, he wrote. Arrogant doctors refused to believe in handwashing, which was promoted and proven effective by Dr. Ignaz Semmelweiss. Yet no one listened. Then, as today, doctors were reluctant to relinquish "their truth." Don't we all suffer from this?

I went, rather dutifully, to college, but medicine was drawing me in by osmosis.

I can still picture my first day walking up Hamilton Walk to the front door of the University of Pennsylvania School of Medicine, the oldest medical school in the United States. I was in awe. We were first going to study anatomy. I was given the prestigious long white coat as we were assigned four to a cadaver. This was experiential learning—hands on is still the best way to gain the knowledge and skills a doctor needs. We were timid at first, barely nicking the skin with our scalpels. Half of each day in our first semester was spent learning muscles, nerves, organs, and all in between. We were allowed to go into the anatomy lab at night to study and dissect. One night I found myself in the lab alone except for thirty cadavers. Spooked at being surrounded by death, I left.

I didn't encounter patients until my second year when we learned physical diagnosis—all the signs of disease from heart murmurs, to lung sounds, to enlarged organs. We were all so timid to be with real live people. In fact, one of my colleagues passed out simply listening to the heart of a pleasant old lady! In the third and fourth years we finally made it to the wards of the hospital and began learning about the care of patients.

During the later years of medical school, we began to make choices. I bonded most with the internal medicine faculty. The Chief of Medicine, Dr. Francis Wood, Sr., often lectured to our class about bedside medicine. One day he brought a patient of his into one of those classic amphitheaters with tiered wooden benches. He taught us a lesson I haven't forgotten.

"Students, today I'm going to present to you a very interesting case."

Our ears perked up, even among those drowsing on the back bench.

"Now I've just made two mistakes. What are they?"

Silence.

"First of all, I've introduced Mrs. Ahrens as a case—not as a person with a name. Why not introduce her by name? Of course

I should have. There's a power differential between doctor and patient. We need to humanize the connection as much as possible."

Then he said, "OK, what other mistake did I make?"

More silence.

"I called Mrs. Ahrens 'interesting.' I suppose that we'd all like to be considered interesting. But an interesting case? I don't think so. In a sense labeling her as "interesting" allies us with her illness—not with her as a person. We need to always consider the person under our care. She is a person placing incredible trust in us."

When I rotated to the surgery service, it was like entering another universe. We had powerful, world class surgeons teaching us, authors of textbooks who possessed almost unlimited arrogance. Every medical student goes through a process of elimination when deciding what kind of doctor they want to become. We heard the old saying: "Internists know everything and do nothing; surgeons know nothing and do everything; psychiatrists know nothing and do nothing; and pathologists know everything and do everything, but it's too late."

We heard that pediatricians wear bow ties, are short, and love to laugh and play; that surgeons are decisive but arrogant; that proceduralists are "scoping for dollars"; that orthopedists have long hairy arms reaching to the floor; and that family doctors are the most balanced. There may be a grain of truth in the medical school palaver, but I think doctors chose their specialties based on experiences during medical school combined with personality and temperament. I decided against pediatrics when my attending shot me with a squirt gun for giving a wrong answer—right at the bedside!

The first case I ever scrubbed in on was an open heart procedure back in 1963. The unfortunate patient had severe aortic stenosis (narrowing of the valve). Having changed into my scrubs, put on my cap, paper booties and scrubbed in, I meekly entered the inner sanctum of the OR. The head nurse spotted me and immediately barked, "Here take this gown, go stand in the corner, and don't do anything until I tell you!"

Other staff came in and one by one put on their gown and gloves. Finally, I was at the side of the operating table, trying to peek around the two residents assisting the thoracic surgeon. One of them made huge incision, inserted a blade much like a small hoe into the cavity, and handed the handle to me. "Here. Keep pulling on this so I can see. Harder!"

After four hours, the operation was done, the bleeding controlled, and the patient sent back to the surgery floor. But almost immediately, problems became apparent. The patient had low blood pressure and a slow heart rate—not good signs. My role as a medical student was to sit by his bedside on the surgical ward overnight and attempt to rescue his falling blood pressure with levophed, a powerful stimulant. But we had neither ventilators nor oxygen monitors, and the patient died at about 3 AM. It was a humbling experience. I knew we were at the limits of available science, and the feelings of powerlessness and fatigue were overwhelming. We weren't counselled about our feelings around death in those days. But I knew that to survive medical school, I'd have to find a way to get through nights like this. To this day, some sixty years later, I still have medical school dreams that border on nightmares.

At autopsy, a fatal mistake was discovered. The wall between the left and right ventricle had been punctured during surgery, not the aortic valve. This meant the heart could no longer effectively function as a pump. I don't know what the surgeon felt. He was the author of the major textbook on thoracic surgery and many research papers. It was in the very early days of heart surgery and it had to start somewhere I suppose, but it didn't make me want to be a pioneer.

After all this, I chose internal medicine and ultimately more training in infectious diseases, pulmonary and critical care medicine. Strangely, the intensity of the ICU isn't that different from the operating room. It is about life and death. But in the OR, there is only one leader. You don't break for a conference or try to reach a team consensus. The surgeon is expected to know what to do, to do it well, and to do it fast (better outcomes with less time under anesthesia). As a nurse said, "The surgeon is like a god in the OR."

But the surgeon is changing. I walked into the ICU to see a post-op consult recently, and asked the woman I assumed to be the nurse her assessment of the patient's vital signs. She smiled and politely corrected me. "I'm the new urologist. We just created an artificial bladder for this patient with bladder cancer." I profusely apologized for my gaff and she let me off gently. Later, at the nurse's desk I asked her to explain the surgery. "It's just sewing," she said. "After removing the bladder, you take a piece of bowel, make a pattern, stitch it all together, plug in the ureters from each kidney, and voila!"

Although you might see why I didn't become a surgeon, I hope you understand that I have great respect and awe for their arduous training, for their skills and stamina, and yes, guts.

I loved my sleep-deprived internship. Being in the hospital, I would see the craziness of the emergency room—the gunshot wounds and the ravages of poorly managed diseases. Losing a patient with asthma was my first experience in an avoidable death. In the ER, an eighteen-year-old had been given too much epinephrine, aminophylline, and phenobarbital—a toxic mix of medications. With him, and other patients, I learned about CPR, using a defibrillator, and how often these heroic efforts fail.

I began to see medical errors and physician burnout. I also saw that hospitals did a poor job of reaching into their communities. The systems were too inward looking to understand. Episodic care for the poor was the norm.

After my residency in internal medicine and a post-doctoral fellowship in infectious diseases, I took a clinical faculty position heading the admitting ward at the local tuberculosis sanatorium. Firland was the major chest referral hospital in Seattle. It was at Firland that I decided pulmonary disease was what really interested me. The lungs bring us the breath of life. It is one of the few organs that are under both voluntary and involuntary control, the interface between the body and the atmosphere, the critical sibling of the heart. So many things were right—or could go wrong—with the lungs.

I accepted a position in internal medicine/pulmonary disease in 1971 with Group Health Cooperative of Puget Sound—now part of the Kaiser Permanente system. The ravages of smoking crowded into my exam rooms. Almost every week there was a new lung cancer and a new patient with emphysema. Ventilators were now common in the ICUs. Medical ethics and end of life decisions were upon us now that we had the technologies of life support. I took additional training in ethics and joined the budding ethics committee, later becoming its co-chair. With the support of a professor, I was able to "grandfather in" and take my pulmonary board certification exam. The exam for critical care was first offered in 1987 and, through experience, I was able to pass that test as well.

As I would come on service in the ICU, I would inherit the care of several patients on ventilators. All too often, the families were struggling with what to do. Frequently there had been no prior communication with their loved ones. I began absorbing the stories around me. I marveled that society gives the medical profession so much trust. We learn your intimate secrets, we examine your bodies, and we try to guide you toward your goals. I learned from social workers about addiction and domestic violence. Nurses taught me about the heroics of caregivers.

When I was a kid, death was just a concept in the distance. Life was ahead, not death. But over time, particularly through my medical practice, death has become a much more pervasive presence. I have seen it manifest in every possible variety—tragic, traumatic, expected, and sometimes as a joyful release. Now at eighty-one, I certainly think more about my own mortality. Yet as I confront the topic—through giving interviews, leading discussions, experiencing the loss of my own friends and family, and writing this book—death no longer frightens me. My hope is that we can all have a good death when our time comes. Strangely, talking and writing about death has brought me a heightened awareness of the life force and potential for joy in living that sustains us all.

THE LESSONS COME HOME

My father was the last of a breed of bedside family physicians. To spend time with him, I'd tag along on his rounds making house calls after dinner. We'd drive to parts of town I'd never seen, using the car's spotlight to search out the right house number—no small difficulty. I'd usually wait in the car as he heaved his rather large and mysterious black doctor's bag out of the car and headed for the front door.

He'd spend about a half hour with each patient. On his return, I'd always ask if he'd given a "shot." Sometimes he had, often a diuretic or vitamin B12.

"Lots of people like their B12," he said.

When I asked why, he shrugged. "I don't know. It's probably just a placebo, something like a sugar pill."

I didn't understand what he meant until years later.

Dad was born in 1907, in Middleport, Ohio, halfway between Pittsburgh and Cincinnati on the banks of the Ohio River. He said he'd learned to swim when some "bully girl" pushed him off the dock. Reminiscent of Huck Finn, he would swim out with friends and float around in the Ohio, only to develop life-threatening typhoid fever at age seventeen. He almost died during that time before antibiotics. His younger brother died of "summer complaint," likely a form of dysentery, at the age of one. Both illnesses would be easily treated with modern medicine.

I was always fascinated by the mystery of what dad really did as a doctor. His office was on the second floor of an old building that he shared with another doctor, though they weren't partners. The visits were inexpensive and mostly small cash payments. He would round on his patients daily in the hospital and essentially was always "on call" except when out of town. Dad loved doing obstetrics so we'd have to plan family vacations around his patients' due dates.

We lived a middle-class existence in a comfortable but far from fancy house in Akron. Dad's friends were specialists who had fancier homes and cars. When, in later years, he finally had enough money to join a golf club, my mother refused to eat there because of the club's discriminatory practices around race and religion.

As dad aged, he decided to drop obstetrics so his practice gradually became geriatrics and nursing home rounding. He kept this up until his mid-seventies. After that he'd make social calls to his patients in the hospital, go to memorial services, and speak at them when families requested. One thing he never forgot to do was send letters of condolence.

But as his prostate began to enlarge and obstruct his bladder, my dad the doctor was curiously reticent about seeking medical care for himself. He'd had both hips replaced in his eighties, but by his nineties ended up in an electric wheelchair, due to crippling spinal stenosis. He lived in a nursing home with several of his former patients. Dad would wheel by, chat, and pat them on the arm. He never quit making rounds, partly because he hated to be alone. Depression was part of the problem and his physician put him on a low-dose anti-depressant that seemed to help. Later, I asked Dad if he was still feeling so low.

After a pause, he said with a wry smile, "No, not really. But I ought to be!"

In his last year as Dad's health declined, my sister Pat moved him to a new nursing home, closer to her home. He was losing weight, so a battery of tests was ordered, including a chest and abdominal CT scan that showed his heart was enlarged (which we already knew). I felt these measures were unnecessary. Why do so much testing on a ninety-three-year-old man nearing the end of his life? Everything came up "normal" except for a tiny, 1 cm spot on his left kidney. Whether this spot indicated a benign or malignant tumor was clinically irrelevant. It wasn't related to his decline. Still, my sister worried. "Shouldn't it be biopsied or removed?"

"Pat, I don't think so," I told her. "Basically, dad is dying. His body is just shutting down."

I had talked with Dad years earlier about his advance directives for end-of-life care. Initially, he was reluctant to sign anything. "They'll just shove me into a corner and not do anything," was his first response to my suggestion that he explicitly state he did not want CPR. I did not give up. I explained how important it was to assign an advocate who could speak for him if he could not speak for himself. Finally, he chose my sister as his durable power of attorney for health care. We talked about palliative care, which would ensure that he felt no pain or discomfort. He decided that he didn't want any heroic measures—such as intubation or CPR—nor did he want to suffer. When we talked about tube feedings he said, "No, when my time's up, my time's up."

After learning that Dad had stopped eating, I flew to Pennsylvania. He recognized me, but it was obvious that he was dying. His voice was raspy, and he was only taking a few sips of liquids. His care at the nursing home was excellent, and the aides very attentive. We set up a bridge table in his spacious room, and I slept there on a cot. We played the music he enjoyed, and family members visited to say their goodbyes. Within a few days, Dad stopped drinking. He gradually slipped into a coma. We used moist mouth swabs to prevent him from getting parched. If he looked at all uncomfortable, a nurse gave him a small dose of morphine.

I'd met with Dad's doctor to advocate for comfort care, which is what Dad always said he wanted. But what if I hadn't intervened? Would the default decision have been to opt mindlessly for more endless interventions and "lifesaving treatment?" How can we ensure that a ninety-three-year-old approaches the end of his life in a dignified manner where his choices are honored?

I spoke to one of the aides as she was going off shift on a Friday. "You know, my father might not be with us when you come back on Monday, "I said.

"Oh, I always have them call me if anything happens to one of my patients."

I was stunned at such an intimate level of caring. How fortunate dad was to be in a small-town nursing home with such a staff. Would that we were all surrounded by people like this at the end.

After four days without fluids, I heard dad take his last breath as I lay on my cot near his bed. I felt him released. His tired old body finally let go, and he was at peace. But I'll never forget my sense of emptiness that early morning.

One relative had objected to the way we handled dad's care. "You're going to take those old people and just let them die?" he said angrily. "Why not give IVs or something?" He felt our society was steeped in a "culture of death."

We listened to him, but I told him that our responsibility was to carry out dad's wishes, which we did. There is a time to let go.

A TIME TO DIE

From time to time, nurses in the ICU would tell me that a dying patient seemed to be clutching at the last threads of life. And as I came into the room of one such patient, I overheard her daughter saying, "Mom it's OK to pass on. Dad is waiting for you. We will all be OK. We love each other as much as we love you." The permission from loved ones to "let go" sometimes seems to be necessary for a patient to exit this life.

But sometimes, patients really take charge. A friend related the story of a revered nun who was dying. The fellow Sisters were gathered around her bed singing and chanting. The nun didn't want any of that. Sitting up she said, "Oh please stop, please leave me alone. Can't you see I'm trying to die?" It was time.

WHAT'S A GOOD DEATH?

Someone once asked a philosopher how he would like to die. He answered: "When I least expect it."

Although many of us may feel the same, we are more likely to age slowly, acquire a few chronic conditions, have periodic illnesses with declining health, and then suffer some kind of "terminal event."

With that pattern in mind, many people ask me, "So what is a good death?" It's a problematic term. What could possibly be good about death? What it really means is a comfortable dying process. I prefer to call it a healing death.

However we feel about our own end of life, or that of a loved one, modern medical technology allows us enough time to think about this idea and what a "good death" for each of us would be. It needn't be an oxymoron.

Death can be healing to caregivers and loved ones left behind when there is a sense that what matters most to a dying person has been honored. When the directives were followed; the health care workers were competent and kind; and hospice and palliative care teams were gracious. When we could all say goodbye.

Understanding the opposite, the pain and difficulty that can mark the last months, or days, of some lives helps bring this into perspective, because even when we are ready to "let go," a battalion of medical technologies may be trying to keep us alive.

Ellen Goodman, Pulitzer Prize-winning author and founder of The Conversation Project, was inspired to confront this after witnessing the experience of her mother's final days. She writes: "The last thing my mom would have wanted was to force me into such bewildering, painful uncertainty about her life and death. I realized only after her death how much easier it would have all been if I heard her voice in my ear as these decisions had to be made. If only we had talked about it."

Yet it is hard to imagine what it will be like for us at death's door. Will it be painful? Will there be shortness of breath? Will we panic, or fear being alone? Will there be regrets? A good death means different things to different people. If we have fears, we want them addressed. If we have preferences for a specific treatment (or non-treatment), we want that honored. What matters most will be unique for each of us. But whatever the particulars, I think each of us wants to be listened to, deeply understood, and comforted with those we love nearby.

A good death is also a nuanced concept. If we climb mountains while knowing we may die in the pursuit, that risk might be worth it to us. If we have terminal cancer and want medical assistance in dying (MAID), that choice could signify a good death. If we are in prison, or in war, those situations will recalibrate notions of a good death. Perhaps our greatest wish is to leave a legacy. The bottom line is that death is personal. It can be thought of as "good" only if it fits with our individual values, and answers our concerns. But how can they be known at the moment of greatest need?

Before the Covid-19 pandemic, the top two leading causes of death for Americans were heart disease and cancer, and they will be so again. However we die, even after a healthy life and good medical care, it is likely that there will be frailty and illness. And it's important to know, beforehand, about the realities of all the choices in front of us.

Do we really understand what it means to be in intensive care, to have our heart shocked by a defibrillator and breathe by use of a ventilator? Invasive treatments can save lives. But they can also prolong the agony of death. Unless we understand these truths—and advocate for our choices about them—there is a good chance that we'll end up on the conveyor belt of ever-increasing medical intervention. When is enough, enough? This is a question each of us must ponder. When is it time to let go?

At some point as we go through the routine of our daily lives, we find ourselves shocked by someone else's death. It enters our minds. We begin to ruminate. What will it be like to die? It is my hope that these thoughts prompt each of us to begin seriously considering our choices, and talking about our wishes with loved ones. Ideally, those conversations lead to a process called advance care planning. Planning for the inevitable is important. It may be the only thing, in the end, that allows us some control over our final days.

There are many sources that can help with this, including guides in English and Spanish to take you step-by-step through preparing your advance directives. I've included my selections in an Appendix at the end of this book.

You may ask: why is this a worthwhile exercise? Can't I just deal with it when my time comes? Most likely, no. Many illnesses progress so rapidly that you may not be able to make your wishes known. This leaves your family or friends guessing, struggling with difficult choices about what to do—use any and all invasive procedures, or not? Keep you alive via ventilator for week? Months?

Without prior discussion, your loved ones will have to use their best judgment about what you might have wanted. And if you're unable to communicate, you can only hope they get it right.

Actually, I don't think these discussions should wait until your waning years. Advance directives are something every adult should have. In a recent lecture I gave to a class of law students, we discussed the issue of tube feeding for Nancy Cruzan, a young woman in a vegetative state after a car accident. Nancy's family wanted her feeding tube removed, but the hospital refused. The young woman had no advance directive. Was the family acting in her best interest? The class of law students in front of me was divided. I asked if any of them had completed their own advance directives. As you might expect, none had. They felt that death was "out there" but not close to them—yet. As with the Cruzan case, some of the following stories involve adults facing death in the prime of their lives.

Whenever it happens, more than half of us will be unable to participate in decisions about our health care in our last two weeks of life. We may be on life support, heavily medicated, or have impaired brain function, all of which impede decision-making capabilities. So who will speak for us? This, unfortunately, was a common situation for patients I tended in the ICU. The social worker and I faced it frequently enough that we eventually developed and published a step-by-step format for discussions with families.[1] If a patient had no advance directives, we'd turn to the spouse or children and develop a community for shared decision making about what their loved one might want in terms of interventional treatment. We tried to learn about the patient's daily life, medical history, and what his wishes might be for various treatments. But of course, we were guessing. We made these decisions without truly knowing.

In summary, the philosophy of advance care planning is that we have the right to direct our care. But we also have responsibilities. We need to understand the benefits and burdens of some of the treatment options and then decide what kind of medical care we would want if we become critically ill. Where would want to be as we die? Who will speak for us if we can't speak for ourselves?

In talking with many patients over the years, I've found there are six aspects that come up for almost everyone in pondering their own "good death."

- Preparation for death—spiritual, emotional and physical needs addressed
- Advance directives—having a strong advocate and clear documents
- Pain and symptom management—palliative care consultation and hospice when needed, without delay
- Completion of goals—each individual has his/her own wishes
- Contributing to others—a legacy
- Being at peace and surrounded by loved ones—most people wish for a home or home-like death.

Your values, indeed your advance care documents, should be discussed with your medical provider, advocate and family well in advance of a crisis. This is not a one-time process. Like a resume, your advance care documents will change with your age, life events, and health status. A good plan evolves from multiple conversations.

A CAT ON THE BED

There's an unusual book, *Making Rounds with Oscar,* about a special, somewhat clairvoyant cat. Dr. David Dosa worked caring for Alzheimer's patients in a Boston nursing home. An uncanny cat, Oscar, appeared to have unfailing accuracy for being able to identify a patient on their last day of life—he would jump on the patient's bed and refuse to leave. No one could determine how he knew when death was imminent.

Dr. Dosa worked mainly with pre-terminal and terminal Alzheimer's patients, and he made a practice of delving deeply into interactions with the family, patient, and staff on every case. For many families, it is difficult to accept that their loved one is dying and that hospice care is the best option at the end. There are endlessly sad stories of families trying to "do everything"—from ventilators to CPR—to keep someone alive, even if their body is trying to shut down.

This brings to mind a patient of mine I'll call Frank. He had severe lung disease and was on oxygen. Every time I brought up end-of-life care Frank got angry. "Listen doctor, I'll decide that when the time comes. I don't want to think about it. And if I'm unconscious, then my kids can decide what needs to be done."

"Frank, have you talked about your wishes with your children?"

"No, but they love me and will know what to do."

A few months later, Frank, severely gasping, called 911 when he couldn't breathe. The medics found him blue, a sign that he wasn't getting enough oxygen, so they put a tube down his throat into his trachea. He struggled so much that they had to sedate him. At the hospital he was placed under my care in the ICU. He had pneumonia that was slow to heal. After about four weeks on a ventilator, during which time he was constantly sedated, it was clear that this was going to be a much longer trial for Frank. We performed a tracheotomy, and kept up with nutrition and muscle strengthening. Attempts to wean Frank off the ventilator were unsuccessful.

During all this, his family struggled terribly. What would Frank really want? Was he in pain? Communication was difficult because when awake he was so agitated that doctors felt they needed to medicate him again. Finally, Frank was sent to a chronic ventilator facility where they specialized in cases like his—trying every means possible to keep him going.

Frank spent two more months there before succumbing to a stroke. His end-of-life wishes remained unknown. It had been impossible for his family to limit care. So, by making no decision, Frank had really decided on the default choice—do everything.

Only a third of adults in the U.S. have advance directives. Recently, I was speaking to a ninety-two-year-old woman and asked about her wishes for something like cardiopulmonary resuscitation (CPR). She replied, "Well, I'll think about it when the time comes, I guess." We must be aware that the norm in our society is to preserve life. If we collapse, a stranger can bare our chest and begin CPR while someone else calls 911. In essence, we are all signed up automatically for heroic life-saving measures unless we explicitly designate otherwise—and do so in a way that is easily discoverable.

When Oscar eventually approaches our bed, we need to be ready. Can we say, "I've lived a full life, told everyone that I love them, apologized to those I needed to, and be at peace? Yes, and now it's time to let go."

Let's hope we can smile when Oscar hops on our bed and snuggles up close.

THE PLAN THAT DIDN'T WORK

I got a call from the ER doc. "Jim I've got a sad situation here. A patient has been brought in by Medic One after having CPR, shocks, and intubation at home. This woman's daughter just arrived and is very upset. Her mom was ready to die."

I was on-call for admissions to the ICU that day, and did not know this patient or her daughter. But I soon learned their story. Susan had advanced cancer and had wanted to die peacefully, in her own home. She had been considering, but had not yet contacted, hospice. A neighbor came by to relieve Susan's daughter, Brenda, just long enough for Brenda to do some shopping.

Just then, Susan moaned and stopped breathing. Not knowing what to do, the neighbor dialed 911. The medics arrived within minutes. The neighbor identified herself as a friend saying, "I'm not sure what type of cancer she has. But I think it's bad."

"Are you related or do you have a power of attorney for health decisions?" the medic asked.

"Well, no."

Not having any instructions to the contrary, the medics performed CPR, placed an endotracheal tube in Susan's airway, and rushed her to our ER, unconscious.

The intake doctor reviewed her records, which revealed she did indeed have a lung cancer that had spread to the bones and brain. A Do Not Resuscitate order had been entered into Susan's chart. On the phone with me he sighed, "None of this should have happened."

Being the physician on call for ICU admissions, I went in and met with Susan's daughter. After conferring with her, we removed the ventilator and let the Susan die in the ER. Social services spent time supporting Brenda and other family now arriving at the hospital. The medics were upset that they'd performed CPR on such a patient. Brenda was furious. And no one in the ER was pleased to have a patient die there, but a hospital admission seemed pointless.

Dying shouldn't happen this way. Better planning might have saved everyone pain and trauma—not least, Susan. There are steps we can take.

Advance care planning is a gift—to ourselves, our loved ones, and our health care team. The first step is to think about values. What matters most to you? What makes life worth living? I advise people to write a short essay about themselves and what the term "acceptable quality of life" means to them, then attach this document to their advance directives. It serves as a framework for working through scenarios you might not have anticipated. You might say, "I do not want to be a burden on my family. I don't want to ever be in such a physical state that my family or someone they hire must care for me 24/7." Or: "I want to breathe naturally and could only accept a ventilator for a short time if my doctor thinks I have a good chance of breathing on my own again. If not, let me die a natural death." Or: "Please do everything possible to keep me alive!"

The next step is the most important. Advance directives cannot address every situation. So we need to discuss our wishes with someone we trust to be our spokesperson when we are unable to speak for ourselves. Someone who will know what we would have wanted, even if it isn't spelled out in the advance directive. Legally, this person is called the "durable power of attorney for health care." They should be someone special to you. Someone who knows your heart, can communicate well, and be a strong advocate—able to stand up to others and speak forcefully for your wishes. They also need to be available—ideally, at the bedside when it counts. This is the person a physician will turn to when weighing critical choices. So it's got to be someone you trust.

In considering treatment choices at the end of life, there are generally three levels of care. First is full life support. This includes all measures to keep a person alive—ventilator, CPR, tube feedings, and such things as dialysis. Anything and everything that will preserve life, no limit. But often, patients and their families don't understand what "do everything" actually means. CPR, for example, can be lifesaving. The way it looks on television would give you the impression it's mostly effective. This is far from the truth. In reality, overall survival rates from a cardiac arrest are around 15%. And when people learn what is involved in CPR, they often gasp. It necessitates pushing down—hard and fast—on a person's chest about one hundred times per minute. The force frequently breaks patients' ribs, especially if they are elderly. For younger people, survival rates are better—as high as 50% when CPR is immediately initiated and the heart tracing shows a "shockable" rhythm. But fewer than one in twenty frail elderly people survive a cardiac arrest long enough to be discharged from a hospital. If they do, the next stop is usually a nursing home.

Tube feeding is another life-saving measure to consider. If you had a severe stroke, would you want to be kept alive by means of a tube? It's a fearful notion for many, the idea of being confined to a bed in a nursing home, unable to move or communicate, clinging to life by means of a tube. Considering that scenario, some people elect to forego artificial feeding if there is little chance of recovery.

Secondly, there is selective care, which is just what it sounds like—some of this, less of that. One could say, for example, it's OK to put me on a ventilator or feeding tube for a few weeks, but I would not want CPR. Or, more commonly, no ventilator or CPR, but I'm ok with being in a hospital for such things as intravenous medication. If you had severe Alzheimer's, would you want an antibiotic? Again, what are your hopes and what are your fears?

Lastly, there is comfort care. This is the most common choice for those with the frailty of old age, end-stage disease and on hospice. The goal is to treat symptoms, knowing there is no cure. Management of pain, emotional distress, shortness of breath, or any other discomfort is the goal. Hospice and this kind of palliative care have brought profound improvements and helped many more people to have a good death. With so many of us living longer, there is an increasing need for physicians trained in this kind of treatment.

Any one of these three options can be selected on a Physician's Orders for Life Sustaining Treatment form, commonly known as the POSLT (or, when referred to as Medical Orders for Life Sustaining Treatment, a MOLST). The POLST was pioneered in Oregon in 1991, and since then has spread. POLSTs are now available, or under development, in all fifty states and Washington DC.

Medicare now covers doctor visits to discuss advance directives and complete these forms. They are most useful for people who want selective or comfort care and wish to forgo CPR and a ventilator. I think of the POLST as "the 911 form." It's just a set of legal orders signed by your health care team and, importantly, by you the patient. It is a bright color—difficult to miss—and very useful in critical situations when 911 is called or an unknown patient arrives in the emergency room. The POLST indicates "go" vs. "no-go" on starting CPR if you're in cardiac arrest.

Your signed POLST forms should be stored in an obvious place for any emergency responders to locate. Assisted living apartments often have a specific designated location. At home, many people keep their POLST form on the refrigerator door or at the foot of the bed. Believe me, medics on emergency calls are grateful to see the POLST form. It helps them know what to do. Some states also allow certified DNR (Do Not Resuscitate) bracelets or medallions, which serve a similar purpose for those who may not have a POLST form with them when they are out and about.

Copies of your advance directives and POLST also need to be given to your advocate, physician, and ideally, scanned into your electronic medical records for access any time.

A POLST form, and hospice, might well have prevented Susan's unfortunate last moments. In the retirement community where I live now, there is a uniform policy. The POLST form, medical history, and current medications are stored in a plastic folder that hangs inside of the door under the kitchen sink. All such residences should do something similar.

WAS IT FUTILE?

I was surprised to get a call from security at SEA-TAC Airport that my patient was being transported by Medic One to our hospital, shortly after touching down. Mary had been insisting on more care for her Stage IV lung cancer and was hoping for a miracle. She'd traveled overseas for what she described as "the miracle cure" so I had lost touch with her over the prior few months. The medics reported that she had shallow breathing and an unstable blood pressure so we admitted her directly to the ICU since she was still "full code" status—that is, "do everything"—per her wishes and written advance directive.

But shortly after arrival at the hospital, Mary's status deteriorated. Her oxygen levels were dropping despite non-invasive support. She was intubated and placed on a ventilator with the usual accompanying measures of tube feeding and close monitoring for complications. Her chest x-ray showed that the tumors in her lungs had grown, spreading to her liver, bones, and brain.

Mary's family was conflicted about the next move. Her husband had had a stroke and was unable to speak, yet he attended our discussions and expressed support for his wife's wishes. But the children, all grown, were divided about the best way to proceed. One wondered if we were only prolonging Mary's suffering. Another felt his mother couldn't have been in her right mind to want invasive treatments that were hopeless—even though she'd specified these wishes in her advance directive.

I was frank with them. Mary, now unconscious, was unlikely to ever get off the ventilator and beyond any hope of recovery. I recommended that the family consider withdrawing ventilator support because it felt like we were prolonging her death, rather than supporting her life. This conversation took place over several meetings, as I tried to introduce the concept of non-beneficial or futile care.

But the family remained conflicted and could not come to a decision. After three weeks in the ICU, Mary's heart stopped and the nurses—against their wishes—performed fruitless CPR. Mary thus died in a needlessly traumatic way.

Futility, medically speaking, is difficult to pinpoint. It remains a concept with which society, and the law, have not fully come to terms. (Thaddeus Pope's excellent blog[2] has frequent posts on the legal issues surrounding end-of-life care and futility.) Generally, this conversation centers on sometimes-conflicting ethics around autonomy, non-maleficence, and beneficence. Debating the limits of each is a healthy thing, and I suspect that every ICU in the country has patients for whom this discussion applies, since 70% of all deaths in the ICU are related to withdrawal of the ventilator—the only thing keeping these patients going.

I believe we will gradually develop better policies around the definition of futility in a medical context. The decision to withdraw ventilator support, even when expected, is never easy, but it often shows respect for the wishes of a patient, as reflected through their advocate. There are times, sadly, when the ventilator is continued for days, weeks, or even months if the decision-makers disagree—but fortunately the futile continuation of care is unusual.

What do we do when a hospital Ethics Committee determines that a patient's care is futile? Simply inform the family that we plan to discontinue ventilator support and allow their loved one's death? In reality, that's very hard to do. Most policies allow families to try finding another institution to provide the treatment they want. But does that solve anything? We once had a patient on a ventilator in our ICU for more than a year because his family was in frequent contact with the press, threatening to "blow the whistle" if ventilator support was withdrawn. This patient was in a vegetative state and subsequently died on the ventilator.

The frustrating bottom line is that too few of the frail elderly have had an informed discussion about the pros and cons of CPR and ventilator support. Even if we decide, "Heck, I'd never want anything like that," a lot can still go wrong in terms of knowing and respecting our wishes. Even a "DNR" or "No Code" tattoo on your chest isn't legally binding![3] So in addition to having "the conversation" with our doctor and loved ones, we need to come up with a written plan.

Do physicians always need consent to write a DNR (Do Not Resuscitate) order? In the U.S., it's ethically questionable for such an order to be written without consent from the patient or their surrogate. In Mary's case, she'd persistently sought a miraculous healing from her lung cancer; hence the search for new therapies in another country, even after top medical care in the U.S. had "failed." With advanced medical technology there is almost always something "more" that we can do. But sometimes, "more" ends up merely prolonging suffering and the dying process.

Ethics Committees vary in their effectiveness from hospital to hospital, and are often underutilized. They don't make clinical decisions, but their review and advisory statements can carry considerable weight. The best of these committees will include patients or their advocates in deliberations, rather than having a closed-door process.

When to stop CPR is an interesting question. In the early days, some hospitals would carry out a foot-dragging "slow code" and allow a terminal patient to die without much trauma. But going through the motions of CPR in this very limited manner was, in my view, entirely unethical.

Between countries, there is considerable difference in ICU end-of-life management.[4] In some, there are limited ICU visiting hours, and if doctors determine that the situation is hopeless, they will extubate the patient—that is, allow him to die with appropriate comfort measures, and then let the family know after the fact. This would never fly in the U.S., where autonomy of the individual is the highest value and often trumps other ethical questions.

The COVID-19 pandemic has brought all of these end-of-life discussions urgently to the fore. During its early days, these conversations[5] often happened in the emergency room to prevent unnecessary CPR and ICU admissions. This can be harrowing for survivors. But it needn't be. With an experienced physician trained in palliative care, patients or their advocates can make these decisions in an atmosphere of caring.

MORAL DISTRESS IN THE ICU

"Doctor, the patient in Room 8 is ready to die, but no one seems to get it except us. Could you please, please talk to the family? It's nuts around here."

Pleas like this were not unusual to hear when I came on for my shift in the ICU. The nurses were like front line troops, sometimes wondering what in the hell the generals were doing, and they frequently unloaded feelings of frustration, sadness, and at times moral outrage at the prolonged care of terminal patients. The hopelessness of the situation was their primary worry, the continued suffering of both a patient and her family. Why couldn't she be allowed to die?

The nurses were not at all cavalier. They had developed these feelings after hours at a patient's bedside doing total body care;

consoling the distressed family; titrating pain medications for comfort without over sedation; listening to specialists consider pushing on with treatments like dialysis for a ninety-year-old; and documenting all of this in the medical records. To them, it seemed so futile, maybe even dishonest. They were carrying out medical orders that they knew weren't going to work.

There has been considerable discussion of moral distress among nurses since the term was codified in 1984 as "the experience of knowing the right thing to do while being in a situation in which it is nearly impossible to do it."[6] Very likely, there is similar undocumented distress among doctors and social workers. I mention it here to give readers some sense of what it's like for the professionals on the other side of their loved one's bed. Many critical care doctors retire early or move laterally into less stressful fields. Among those who remain, burnout surfaces in a number of ways. I know a doctor who divorced his first wife to marry an ICU nurse, divorced her to marry a second ICU nurse, and then finally left the ICU altogether for work in a limited practice.

Finally, medicine is devoting more attention to the issue of moral distress and its corollary, moral resilience, on medical frontlines.[7] The idea is to promote environments where people feel empowered to speak up without fear. But likely there will always be situations where hospital staff feel obligated to continue providing care that they find questionable. In our ICU, a social worker met frequently with the nursing staff to help them process the anguish of medical futility and the difficulties of negotiating with a hostile or dysfunctional family.

For my own part, I tried to lighten the atmosphere with gallows humor. "Let me put on my black cape and make rounds with you," I'd say, trying to provoke a laugh among the nurses. They knew I was more willing than some physicians to explain to a family that their loved one was indeed dying. Often, the atmosphere on our rounds was tense, and this kind of banter often helped to relieve the stress.

DYING AT HOME—AN IDEAL
CONTRASTED WITH REALITY

When giving talks, one point I make is that most Americans prefer to die at home or at least in a home-like environment. Bob raised his hand and said, "Not me!" He was in the minority. But he adamantly did not want to die at home. I met with him later to learn his story.

It all started when he had trouble swallowing. Liquids went down fine, but a piece of meat seemed to get stuck. His GI specialist recommended an endoscopy to look at Bob's esophagus. He reluctantly agreed, as long as he could be sedated. The procedure went smoothly, but the pictures showed a rough and angry narrowed area that restricted the passage of food. The diagnosis proven by biopsy was cancer. That was three years ago.

In a subsequent surgery, a large part of Bob's esophagus had been removed and bridged with a portion of his colon. That too, worked fine for a while, but the cancer came back with a vengeance. Chemotherapy and radiation slowed it down temporarily but Bob's treatment options were now exhausted. The cancer was running its course.

Bob was ninety. He had to force himself to eat and was losing weight. He'd developed a hacking cough because liquid intermittently got into his lungs. He knew that pneumonia was a real threat, and that his time was limited. But Bob didn't want to die at home.

"Listen, Doc, I just don't want to have my wife and children watch me die. It's too much of a burden for them. Also, no one wants to buy a house where someone just passed."

Bob was now enrolled with hospice, which was home focused. He loved the nurses, and they had agreed to move him to an inpatient unit at the end, although he was still skeptical about that actually happening. He had standing orders in a POLST form that both he and his doctor had signed. He didn't want CPR, but did want aggressive management of pain and shortness of breath. He was ambivalent about fluids, but did not want a feeding tube. He was worried that if he died suddenly when away from the house, Medic One would be called and CPR attempted. To deal with this, his wife copied the POLST form and carried it with them whenever they left home.

The fact is, dying at home surrounded by loved ones is a somewhat romanticized ideal. Between total body care, sleep deprivation, and medication schedules, the final days of dying can be difficult, with extreme stress on both patient and caregivers. My sister Julie is an example.

JULIE AT HOME

Julie's life had been one medical disaster after another: she had a son with cerebral palsy from a botched birth; paralysis from a drug used for depression; failed low back fusions; a bowel rupture from colitis; and pelvic and shoulder fractures from several falls. But Julie had refused to move to an assisted care facility. She wanted to stay and die in her lovely, impractical, Pennsylvania farmhouse, built in the early 1800s.

Her children and neighbors made this arrangement possible until a stroke landed Julie in the hospital. She had been clear in her advance directives that she did not want CPR or artificial feeding. But in the rush to get her care, these directives were overlooked, and a doctor had placed a feeding tube directly into her stomach through the abdominal wall. It was a screw up, and created enormous turmoil for Julie's family. In general, it is routine for hospitals to ask about advance directives on a patient's admission. But the only way to be sure they are followed, is for our advocates to be on hand with the proper documents.

The hospital advised Julie's family to place her in a skilled nursing facility where she could get physical and occupational therapy. But Julie was insistent.

"No, just send me home. I'm ready to die. I don't want to live like this," she said. Honoring her wishes in this way placed a heavy burden on Julie's family. But they respected her wishes.

So she entered a home hospice program. Julie's three children, my two nephews and niece, learned the twenty-four-hour routine of administering her pain medications, sedation, and body care. But it was wearing. None of them had a medical background, and one felt that the feeding tube should be used. Though the other two disagreed, Julie's son gave her a tube feeding formula during his shift. She was being starved, he thought. Pretty soon, I was getting cross-country phone calls seeking support and direction. My advice was to get more help at home. The stress they were shouldering was just too much.

Worn out, Julie's children finally hired home care aides. There are hospice houses and nursing units for severe issues, but Julie did not wish to be moved. Inpatient hospice beds are limited anyway, so hospice deaths most commonly occur at home, typically with spouses or children as caregivers. This has its challenges. But hospice nurses train and help to support the family caregivers, finding additional aides or other resources as needed.

After three weeks, Julie managed to die peacefully. Later, when I spoke with her family, it became clear that all of this would have been much easier for Julie's children if she'd spent her final days in a nursing hospice unit—yet they respected her wish to die in her beloved home.

Medicare promotes home-based hospice as a cost-effective program, and for most cases it's ideal. Reality, however, is that many patients are referred to hospice so late that they die in just a few days. This is exactly what had happened with Julie's husband, a physician, a few years before her death. He had been hospitalized with cancer, and Julie called me, panicked, when he was discharged though still very ill. Hospice arrived at their home later that day. But the arrangements were chaotic, and he died within twenty-four hours.

Hospice workers want time to get to know their patients' families in order to outline a plan for care. But too often, hospice is delayed because the patient or their family—or even their doctor—perceive it as giving up. Admittedly, for a physician it can be difficult to shift from a curative mindset to palliative care. But, ironically, patients admitted into hospice early sometimes live longer than expected—on rare occasions even improving enough to be discharged. Overall, modern hospice is well-loved by patients and their caregivers, allowing more of us to have a peaceful, family-centered death at home. In fact, in 2017 home as the site of death became more common in the U.S. than in acute care hospitals for the first time.[8] For all of us with life-threatening illnesses, think hospice. And think about it early.

INCURABLE CANCER, BUT NOT FOR MIKE

Mike was a runner and fitness nut. He enjoyed the runner's high and hoped that his athletic lifestyle would help him avoid serious illness. But in his 50s, Mike began to notice blood streaks in his stools, and he also had cramping in his belly. It was a month before he could be scheduled for a colonoscopy. The results were shocking. "There's a cancer in the bowel," Mike's doctor said. "You need an abdominal CT scan ASAP." The scan brought even more serious news. "Mike, the cancer has spread to your lymph nodes, liver, and lungs. It's an advanced—Stage IV."

Mike's wife, Jan, who was present for this conversation, felt like the room was spinning. "Am I really hearing this? Can it be—he's only fifty-three! Could there a mistake? Will he suffer? Is it terminal? How long does he have?"

Mike held a PhD in mathematics and had just won tenure at his university. By nature, he was analytical. Things needed to make sense, including his own health. There were logical ways to deal with all problems. Jan, who had a graduate degree in engineering, looked at life much the same way. Between their jobs, four children, and family life, everything seemed so good. How could this be happening?

Both Mike and Jan jumped on the phone and began calling their academic and physician friends around the country. They scoured the internet for colon cancer treatments, but the findings were grim. Median survival time for colon cancer is about two years after diagnosis. Still, their doctor friends had recommended sources for expert care.

First, they went the conventional route, chemotherapy, hoping this would decrease the size of Mike's tumor. But the side effects of weakness, nausea, and loss of appetite discouraged them.

One of their physician contacts felt they might do better with the more holistic approach offered by a specialized center for cancer care in the southwest. This treatment program involved intravenous vitamins, nutritional supplements, massage, homeopathy, and tai chi in combination with standard chemotherapy. The center staff reassured Mike and Jan that with these "specialized tailored cancer treatments" Stage IV colon cancer did not have to be a terminal disease.

Multiple CT scans and blood tests followed. The tumor shrank but did not resolve, so Mike and Jan got another referral, this time to a West Coast surgeon who would try to "debulk" the tumor by removing part of Mike's colon and liver. The procedure was complicated by a blood clot in Mike's left leg, a piece of which broke off and traveled to his lungs, further complicating the operation. That necessitated anticoagulation treatment and a filter placed in the inferior vena cava to prevent further clots from traveling to Mike's lungs.

By this point, standard treatment options had pretty much been exhausted, yet the tumors kept growing. Another physician friend sent Mike to a research scientist who was aware of drugs "in the pipeline" for cancer treatment, but not available in the U.S. Mike traveled out of the country to receive two of these drugs, one of which was injected directly into his tumors. These "off-label" treatments caused chills, pain, and weakness, but also gave him a transient sense of hope.

Mike's insurance covered only some of these procedures, and he kept tabs on the costs. His trips to the southwest center, off-shore treatments, and alternative doctors totaled $260,000. Insurance paid an additional $290,000 for most of the conventional cancer surgeries, but denied some claims.

In Mike's case, cost wasn't the major issue. It was unrealistic expectations. Mike and Jan had been told at the holistic center that his cancer was curable—if only they could find the right treatments, sending them on a months-long quest. There were prayers, hopes, and an endless cycle of emotional ups and downs for Mike's family and close friends. Well-meaning folks sent them promises of still more miraculous cancer centers, breakthrough treatments, and alternatives. It seemed, always, that the answer was out there if they could just find the right person.

I became aware of Mike's story through his on-line postings, and I felt compelled to talk to him about hospice. He was suffering and dying. So, through mutual friends, I reached out and called him.

"Mike I'm so distressed about your illness and can certainly understand your attempts at seeking out a cure," I said.

"Thanks Jim, I'm still fighting on. I'm too young to die."

"Well, ok. But you might benefit from aggressive treatment of your symptoms by a palliative care team and maybe a hospice consult."

"No way, Jim. I'm not ready to let go."

The end came swiftly. Mike had lost fifty pounds. He was jaundiced and not eating. But hospice still wasn't involved. His children had been bewildered but supportive caregivers, staying in their parents' home to help as much as possible. One morning, Mike awoke in severe pain. His chest was heaving and his breathing hurt. Most of the family was nearby and raced to be at his bedside. There was a flurry of phone calls to hospice and their primary doctor, who told Jan that Mike was dying, likely in a matter of hours. Hospice never made it. Mike slipped into coma and died thirty minutes later.

Although he'd had lots of care, I don't think Mike was well served by his medical providers. His wife and children did their absolute best. But the problem was his wish for a miracle, fed by less-than-honest messages from some doctors. Mike's family, understandably, wanted to hear good news, so they hung on every promise. I don't fault patients seeking out second or third opinions, but the quest for a cure sometimes knows no bounds. I once had a patient with inoperable cancer go to a developing country for "bloodless surgery." My patient returned with photographs of the organs that had been supposedly removed, though there was no scar. They were convinced of the cure, nonetheless. Some "miraculous" cancer treatments have turned out to be injections of normal body substances like creatinine. Cortisone, which gives short term euphoria, is also part of many "alternative cures."

Mike's story isn't unusual. Our society expends huge sums on rather futile care. We want the best for ourselves and are willing to pay for it. But is this rational? At what point should Mike's physician friends have lovingly advised hospice? Mike lived for only fifteen months after his diagnosis, rather than the median of twenty-four. (New chemotherapy and immunotherapy have lengthened the median survival for Stage IV colon cancer up to twenty-nine months, and about nine percent of those patients can live for more than five years.) Is it possible that some of Mike's alternative treatments actually hastened his demise? Even if not, did any of them benefit the quality of his remaining life? I think Mike's case shows how hard it is for us to switch from a curative to a palliative mindset—even among well-meaning, medically knowledgeable people. It also shows how false hopes can contribute to delays in calling hospice. In this case, Mike, Jan and all of their friends were in denial.

A HEALING DEATH

Pete and I both had prostate cancer diagnosed at about the same time. It was difficult to choose what to do, but we both elected surgery. Mine was easy. Pete's wasn't. His cancer had already spread so the surgeons did a wide exploration, removing as much tumor as possible. Then, over the next months, Pete took drugs to block testosterone. But his PSA kept rising, so he started chemo. After two months of this therapy, Pete looked terrible and was admitted to the ICU for severe electrolyte imbalance. Once home again, he sat in a reclining chair that he never left except for trips to the bathroom. One day, over the backyard fence, Lucy let me know how badly Pete had deteriorated. I made a visit. In their living room, I found Pete pale and clammy with a pulse (which I surreptitiously checked) of 130.

Outside, I asked Lucy, "What's the plan if Pete's condition becomes critical?"

"Well, he doesn't want to be resuscitated so I won't call 911," she said.

"Have you contacted hospice yet?"

"None of the doctors have mentioned hospice."

This didn't surprise me. Doctors start off on a curative path and find it difficult to acknowledge that a patient is dying. It can be hard to step back and simply allow death to take its course. The patient and family are often ready for that shift before their doctors. In Pete's case, no one was talking about the elephant in the room.

So I said, "Lucy, please call your doctor and hospice—soon." I brought over a POLST form and told her, "You really need to discuss this with Pete and his medical team."

Hospice arrived the following day. They set up a hospital bed and commode. The family became caregivers, and within a week Pete died. But I could not help wondering how Lucy would have proceeded without an informed advocate.

At Pete's memorial I asked his son, Don, how the family was doing.

"Pretty much OK," Don said, and then he recounted this story: Don and his father had gone for a drive when Pete was still able, and they talked about his dying.

"Dad said, 'Listen, dying is easy for me—I'll just be gone—but I'll need you to help hold the family together. I don't want you to grieve a long time. I'll be OK wherever the Lord takes me. You're a good person, and your mom and sisters too. Things will be all right. Make my memorial a joyful celebration. It's for you all, not for me.'"

As I listened to Don recounting this conversation with his dad, I felt I could see Pete trying to put his impending death into perspective. He didn't want anything left unsaid, and he didn't want his family to worry. He was, in this way, caring for his care-givers and trying to make his death an occasion for healing, rather than unbroken suffering.

As we are dying and beginning to shed our physical connec-tions, we naturally worry about those left behind. But by connect-ing with them, talking, and planning for the end, our death can, counterintuitively, become restorative—healing for our survivors, and for us as well. There is a passing of the torch. This is what Don had experienced in the conversation with his father. I thought of him as the kid I'd once coached in baseball. Now, suddenly, Don was a man—perhaps even more so with the death of his father. Out of death come these new roles, new responsibilities—dare I say it, new life.

If we can accept this, there is the possibility of a healing death. While we may never truly "get over" the loss, a healing death helps lead us toward resilience and the sense that the les-sons of life and love that have been passed on can help us move forward.

That is not always possible, of course. Sometimes death is vio-lent, unexpected, isolated, or full of psychological trauma. I think of the anguish I read in the words of a Black friend who wrote to me during the early days of the COVID-19 pandemic. Her com-munity was suffering disproportionately and, often, alone, with middle-aged people dying unexpectedly and without any hugs, handholding, or bedside vigils. These deaths were medicalized and distant, and in their wake left so many questions unanswered, which is perhaps the most painful part of all.

Different cultures have their own rites and rituals around dying, and even grieving. A healing death must be defined through those terms. Some faiths hold that embalming is wrong, and the body must be buried within three days. For others, scattering ashes in a special place will be the final goodbye. But all of us crave this sense of peaceful completion that comes through respecting a loved one's final wishes.

A NOTE FROM ISRAEL

The struggles faced by families of dying people in the U.S. are not unique to our health care system. An Israeli physician wrote to me to share her own experience, and with her permission I've included it here. It demonstrates two things: 1) How a doctor handled the imminent death of her own parent. (2) The fact that medical professionals face the same battles and quandaries as anyone else regarding jurisdiction around end-of-life issues.

At the center of this story is the question of elder care facilities wanting to hurry dying patients into hospitals. Some nursing homes may be understaffed; or they may not want to report any deaths at their institutions. Perhaps they worry about lawsuits from grieving families. Or maybe they just want to take the path of least resistance—call 911 and then the patient is someone else's problem.

Bottom line: I wish all elderly people had an advocate like Dr. L.

From Dr. L: *I am a family physician in a Kibbutz in Israel, and I take care of almost all the people in the Kibbutz, from birth to death. I am faced with end of life issues quite often.... I am fortunate to be able to help many patients and families to avoid futile hospital care, and this is one of the things I am very proud of.*

A few months ago I took care of my stepfather who lived in a fancy place for old people who can take care of themselves and live alone in a nice flat, but they have a restaurant, have cultural activities etc., in a big city. (I don't know what this kind of place is called in English—here it's called something like "sheltered living.") At the age of 89, he started getting weaker and needed more and more help with his daily activities, until finally he needed constant care. Cancer was diagnosed. We got someone to take care of him 24 hours a day. When he got to the stage where he needed a wheelchair, the management of this place did whatever they could to get him to leave—to a nursing home (with four people in a room), a hospital or whatever. He had already sold his previous home, and he'd expected to live in this place for the rest of his life.

He was alert and understood they wanted to get rid of him, as this spoiled their nice place for "the young at heart." They referred me to the contract where it says that this is a place for independent people. I managed to take care of him in his flat and refused to take him to the hospital, as this was his explicit wish, and we all knew that there was nothing they could do better in the hospital than we could do in his own home and bed. In the last week of his life I was there most of the time, gave him medications against pain, and he passed away in his bed surrounded by those who loved him.

I was very happy to have been able to do this for him. I was very sad that this had to be done fighting the management all the way. They threatened me that I was denying him adequate care in a hospital, where he should be in his situation. I ignored them as I knew his time was getting short, and I didn't believe they would try to evacuate him forcefully in his situation. He passed away a day before another meeting they set up to tell me I had to take him somewhere else.

I am glad to read your stories that show me that I am not alone in the thought that if there is nothing more medicine can do, the best place for a person to finish his life is in his own home, if this is what he wants."

EVERYONE NEEDS AN ADVOCATE

Once a doctor or nurse, always a doctor or nurse, even in retirement. I still get "curbside consult" requests from family and friends. This is normal and expected. But sometimes requests can be problematic: "My son's going to Africa—can you write a prescription to prevent malaria? I have this cough, and the doctor isn't doing anything. What should I do now? Do you think I really need to have this prostate cancer surgery?"

I'm honored to be asked, though I try not to be intrusive. Mostly, I offer questions for them to pose to their own physicians. Sometimes, however, I can't stand by. As the following story makes clear, sometimes I need to step in and advocate.

My sister Pat, who lived in rural Pennsylvania, developed severe shortness of breath. Asthma was the diagnosis, but inhalers didn't help her much. Pat was known to have a leaky heart valve, though it had been stable since childhood when she likely had rheumatic fever. Her primary care doctor referred her to a local cardiologist, who told her she needed three heart valves replaced. Well, at age seventy, nobody needs three new heart valves. This was so over the top that I "interfered" by advising her to get assessed at the Cleveland Clinic, which wasn't too far away.

My sister made the two-and-a-half-hour drive, only to find that her records hadn't arrived so she needed to make yet another trip. Pat described the cardiology consultant as a disengaged "cold fish." He told her no surgery was indicated, nor did he see any need for further tests. Pat was simply too fat, he said. I knew my sister was overweight, but her shortness of breath was more than would be expected, even with that precondition. I worried that something else was going on.

So I stepped in again. I was able to find a pulmonologist at the University of Pittsburgh Medical Center who agreed to evaluate Pat. Doctors don't often relish being the third consultant—basically a referee between two parties of diverging opinion. But he did this for me as a colleague, analyzing Pat's pulmonary functions, CT scans, and cardiac ultrasounds in addition to a careful physical exam. It revealed widespread "crackles" in both lungs—inflamed tissue that sounds like Rice Krispies when a patient breathes. The discovery of these crackles led to a lung biopsy that showed serious, irreversible lung disease—pulmonary fibrosis.

I checked in with Pat by phone every few weeks. She'd tried steroids and other treatments, but her breathing did not improve. I helped her find hospice care, but the hospice base was forty miles away so several different RNs were assigned, which made it difficult to coordinate Pat's care. A regimen of sedatives and narcotics to treat her shortness of breath made her goofy and unstable, and she was finally admitted to an in-patient hospice unit, but only for a week.

After coming home, Pat casually mentioned that she felt hyper and shaky so I reviewed her medications. She was using both long-acting and short-acting asthma inhalers—overdosing, basically. I told her to stop the daily albuterol and use it only as needed. Pat's jitters resolved. I wondered if her team was really on top of things. Too many medications are a common problem when multiple providers are involved.

Then one of her sons contacted me, worried. He'd done an internet search and wondered if Pat's use of oxygen could be toxic. I spent some time reassuring him that in her case, it was fine. But what all of this back-and-forth demonstrates is how badly my poor sister needed an advocate to navigate the messy business of illness and dying.

By this point, Pat had become essentially bedridden. She was on continuous oxygen, though at peace. She believed she would pass into a vibrant, spiritual world in a disease-free spiritual body. While reluctant to leave her husband and family, Pat was actually looking forward to the day when everyone could be together once more.

Weeks later, I received a phone call late at night from Pat's husband. My sister was having a severe nose bleed, he said. They'd already called a nurse and applied cold packs, but the bleeding wouldn't slow. Then Pat came on the phone. "Jim, I really don't want to go to the emergency room. Is it illegal for me to die from a nose bleed?"

I was taken aback. To buy some time and figure out an answer, I asked, "Are you taking any kind of blood thinner?"

"Well, not really. Just my baby aspirin."

I was stunned at this disclosure. Why was a hospice patient being treated with aspirin to prevent a heart attack? Was anyone on her team overseeing Pat's total care? Fortunately, the bleeding stopped without a trip to the emergency room. And I was never pushed to directly answer Pat's question. But no, it's not illegal to die from a nose bleed. We all have the right to control what's done to our bodies, particularly at the time of death.

Doctors are generally advised not to provide care for their own families. There's potential for getting emotionally involved and losing one's clinical detachment. In fact, the pharmacy at my clinic wouldn't fill a prescription for anyone in my family if I wrote it. (This is a marked contrast to days gone by, when my dad used to look at our sore throats and give us shots of penicillin as needed.) From time to time, I have provided care for my own family, stitching up my son's laceration at a Boy Scout Camp when I was the doctor there. (Now a lawyer, he still points to the jagged scar on his knee and says, "Boy, you can sure tell that wasn't done by a plastic surgeon!")

But there are ridiculous extremes. When I was a medical student in 1963, an elegantly dressed surgeon wearing a tailored suit and silk tie lectured our class. "Gentlemen," he said, ignoring the few women in the room, "my wife had severe ulcer disease and needed surgery. I felt the best surgeon was needed, so I decided to do the procedure myself, and she had an excellent recovery." He suffered from what I call MDeity Syndrome.

The primary exception to this rule against providing medical care to a family member is in the instance of assigning an advocate for the end of life.

As I've indicated, finding a strong advocate is perhaps the most important thing we can do to ensure that our wishes are honored at the end. Your advocate can be any trusted person, most commonly your spouse or child. And you should legally designate them as your durable power of attorney for health care. That way, they will be empowered to speak for you when you can no longer advocate for yourself—a common situation in the last weeks of life.

Pat died peacefully at home, her wishes thankfully fulfilled. Morphine relieved her shortness of breath. Her husband and family ministered to her. They had been forceful advocates, continuing to push for more opinions when things weren't going well.

In this sense, Pat was fortunate. Many others spend their final days in nursing homes. States have begun to recognize the need for protection of residents in long-term care, especially those who are homeless, frail, or otherwise disadvantaged. Often these people are isolated and do not understand their rights. In nursing homes, memory care facilities, and adult family homes all patients should have access to a state-sponsored ombudsman, who can act as an advocate.

WHAT ARE OUR RIGHTS IN NURSING HOMES?

I looped my ombudsman's badge around my neck, signed in, and took the elevator to the fourth floor to survey conditions for the residents of a long-term care facility for the elderly in Seattle. I had not announced my visit ahead of time, but now let the executive director and head nurse know I was dropping in to chat with residents. I was there as an outside advocate in this skilled nursing unit which had some very sick long-term patients.

I introduced myself to one of them, Catherine, and explained that I was there to ensure that her care—and that of all the residents—met state requirements. Still, it took a while to break the ice. Mainly, I was there to deal with low-level problems that had been left unresolved. Sometimes that meant complaints about food quality or delayed medication. But Catherine wanted to talk about her wound care. She had an open, deep-pressure ulcer on her lower back and buttocks that wasn't healing. Also, she said her fingers sometimes cramped spasmodically, and she didn't know why. I wasn't immediately aware of any other medical problems, but I could see immediately that she was obese.

After I retired from practice, I decided to learn just what went on in long-term care. Many of my patients went for rehab treatments at Skilled Nursing Facilities (SNFs), but I knew little about day-to-day life in these places. So I decided to volunteer as a long-term care ombudsman. After twelve all-day training sessions, I started visiting nursing home residents a few times a week, listening to them as an advocate.

Catherine signed a waiver allowing me to review her medical records, which were voluminous. She had severe congestive heart failure, diabetes, and poor circulation. Her blood work showed low levels of magnesium, which may have been causing her muscle spasms. But what alarmed me most was her "full code" status. That meant if her heart stopped, Catherine would be intubated, transferred to a hospital, and placed on a ventilator in the ICU. Medically, this made no sense. With so many severe medical problems, she would never survive heroic critical care.

In my role as an ombudsman, it was often difficult to separate my work as an advocate with my experience as a physician. I had to decide how to work with Catherine and her husband to advocate for her care. I asked for permission to speak with Catherine's doctor, inquiring about her low magnesium levels and whether that might be causing her finger spasms. Then I asked about the wisdom of using CPR on a patient like this. My nudge seemed to make a difference. Catherine's doctor began prescribing her magnesium supplements and tried to discuss end-of-life issues with her. But he never wrote a Do Not Resuscitate (DNR) order. There could have been a variety of reasons for that: perhaps Catherine's poor prognosis was never made clear to her; perhaps she didn't understand CPR and ventilators; or perhaps it was just too difficult for Catherine to acknowledge the fact she was dying.

It was frustrating. I knew it wasn't my role to prompt end-of-life discussions with Catherine and her husband. I wasn't her doctor. But I continued to meet with the two of them during my bi-weekly visits to the nursing home. Over the next two months Catherine's condition seemed to worsen. Her legs grew swollen. Her wounds did not heal, and she became increasingly discouraged.

One day, I popped into Catherine's room to say hello—and she was gone. I learned that she'd developed a fever and that her blood pressure had dropped, so they sent her to a nearby hospital. With no small difficulty, I located her room there and was headed in to see her when I saw the "no visitors" sign. Luckily, a medical resident was just leaving Catherine's room, and I buttonholed her, explaining who I was. She said it was OK for me to go in, but cautioned that Catherine was pretty far gone.

"As a colleague," I asked, "can you tell me if you plan to do CPR?"

"No, she's been DNR and DNI since admission."

That meant Do Not Resuscitate and Do Not Intubate. Somehow, this acute care hospital had addressed Catherine's end-of-life questions wishes better than her own long-term facility. Likely, the hospital physicians had spent more time presenting a realistic picture of CPR and ventilators. And once Catherine finally understood, her wishes were clear—no heroic intervention.

I sat at her bedside a few moments and tried to provide some support to her husband, who was also there. A few days later, Catherine died peacefully and comfortably. Her hospital team had consulted with palliative care physicians and provided comfort care with low dose morphine and sedatives.

It takes effort to have meaningful end-of-life discussions. It requires listening, learning, teaching, and willingness to take time out of a busy day. It's often the elephant in the room, the looming question that no one is willing to confront. During Catherine's months in the nursing home, the primary aim was stabilizing her health with expert wound care, a special air bed, antibiotics, nutrition, and good general care. There hadn't been any acknowledgement that plans had to be made, as she was near death.

This is all too common. Nursing homes must abide by a long list of regulations—"Heck, we're more regulated than the nuclear industry," one administrator told me—but providing help to navigate end-of-life questions is not among them. And in my experience, despite the annual reviews and mandatory reports, some long-term care facilities continue to fly under the radar.

Still, there is indeed a long list of protections for residents, few of which are common knowledge. Even as a doctor who frequently treated the elderly, I was largely ignorant of these regulations before my work as an ombudsman. For example, Washington state law[9] says residents are entitled to safe, clean, comfortable home-like environments; notice of their rights and facility policies; disclosure of all fees; an understanding of plans for care; and privacy and confidentiality. There are rights pertaining to residents' transfer or discharge; rights for having grievances addressed; control over funds and financial affairs; protection from chemical or physical restraints; personal property safeguards; privacy of mail and phone calls (meaning no opening letters or listening in); privacy for visits; and no requirement to sign any waiver releasing a facility from liability for losses of personal property or injury.

But who makes sure those rules are abided by? Very often, residents are frail and somewhat befuddled by all the paperwork. "Why are there so many forms to sign?" they may wonder. "I don't understand what's going on. They say I'll be billed even though I have my Medicaid application filed."

Serious incidents require mandatory reporting to the state. But I am skeptical about how often that occurs. As a volunteer, I heard one resident complain of verbal abuse by a night aide; another told me about a fall from her bed; another was inappropriately threatened with a huge bill. (This is a common trick, aimed at encouraging residents to move out when they are transitioning to Medicaid.) The state tries to protect residents through reports and inspections by certification teams. But the number of inspections and case workers is limited, and when problems are discovered I don't have great confidence in the interventions.

The quality of care varies widely. Once, when reporting an incident to a county nurse administrator, I mentioned that the facility must be pretty good because of its five-star rating. "Those ratings don't mean shit!" the nurse said. "Half the time they don't report incidents or find ways to cover things up."

When I was a practicing physician, my own patients usually wanted to stay out of nursing facilities altogether, hoping they could be cared for at home when the time came. But that's not always possible. For some, as I've shown, remaining at home can be isolating for patients, exhausting for caregivers, and even unsafe. Either way, long-term care is a growth industry. There are currently 1.4 million Americans in nursing homes, and that number is only growing. The funding and design of care for the "silver tsunami" of aging seniors remains a serious problem for our nation and many others around the world.

LEARNING TO LISTEN

*T*he most important characteristic of a good doctor is first to be a good listener. The most important part of an office encounter is to understand the patient's story. Everything else follows naturally.

CAN WE HAVE A CONVERSATION?

In the 1960s, when I was in medical school at the University of Pennsylvania, we only whispered about death and dying. An eminent surgeon lectured us, "Students, never tell a patient that they have cancer. Talk to the family, and they will decide what to do." As a student on the surgical service, I vividly recall seeing a patient who'd been referred to a professor of surgery in his private clinic. This elderly woman had advanced breast cancer that had been neglected and was obviously widespread. For whatever reason, she had put off dealing with the reality of her disease and was now consulting with this renowned doctor, desperately looking for hope. He held her hand and said, most disingenuously, "My dear, thank goodness you got to me in time."

Personally, I was shocked. This eminent physician was only perpetuating the patient's avoidance of reality. False hope was the salve this doctor offered. I knew it was wrong, but as a student I could say nothing. Yes, the truth could be cruel. But so can secrets.

Years later, I learned that it is possible to be both caring and direct when dealing with discouraging news. Even in a hopeless situation, doctors should be honest. But I don't think we should ever say "There's nothing more we can do." Because, in fact, medicine can offer care, even when there is no cure.

Talking about death and dying has been taboo in our society, but that is finally changing. A friend in Portland wrote to me that he'd recently attended a Death Cafe[1] a group of strangers who met up at a coffee house to talk about death and dying. He was impressed with the breadth of their discussion about caregiving, making choices, grief, and spirituality. I had heard about this worldwide movement and was skeptical that random people in a meet-up group could have a meaningful discussion about such a personal topic. But my friend's experience helped me to see the value of even relative strangers gaining insight about death through these gatherings.

At the University of Washington there is something similar. Michael Heeb has developed a web site[2] and accompanying book, *Let's Have Dinner and Talk about Death,* to promote conversations over the dinner table. Syndicated columnist Ellen Goodman is also promoting more forthright conversations about death, motivated by the painful experience of her mother's passing. The organization Prepare for Your Care[3] is another useful site that can help us to get started thinking about life's end.

For all these efforts, significant barriers to a forthright approach remain. A few years ago, I attended a lecture given by health care writer T.R. Reid, who was describing different approaches to medical treatment around the world and the shortcomings of our system in the United States. Afterward, I approached Reid, the author of several books, and asked if he'd ever considered writing one about the American style of dying and its excessive costs. Too difficult, he told me. His own family became emotional whenever he tried to bring up the topic.

IT LASTED UNTIL THE END

I always looked forward to Harold's visits. Harold knew that he had life threatening pulmonary fibrosis. He also knew that doctors didn't have the faintest idea what was causing this, even though they used rather toxic medications to keep it under control. Prednisone seemed to work best.

Somehow, Harold forgave me for all the shortcomings of medical science. He liked to chat about his life during office visits: his grandson playing football at Notre Dame; his granddaughter who loved soccer; the holiday celebrations that were special in his family. Over time I thought I had gotten to know Harold pretty well. But did I, really?

He would come in cheerful and bubbling, with a tendency to wave off such symptoms as shortness of breath. But his lungs were progressively filling with scar tissue, which blocked oxygen from getting into his blood effectively. A portable oxygen system helped, and Harold accepted it with grace. With his wife present we had some serious discussions about end-of-life questions, and he had completed an advance directive affirming that did not want to be placed on a breathing machine unless doctors were confident he could return to a meaningful existence. His wife would be in charge if he was unable to make decisions.

One day, during a routine visit in the office, I noted that Harold's severe lung dysfunction had been quite stable for more than a year. "Harold," I said casually, "you know you're really lucky to still be alive." I meant to be encouraging, but my patient burst into tears.

"What's going on," I said rather helplessly. "Did I say something wrong?"

"You don't know how lucky I really am to be alive."

"What do you mean?"

"I was a paratrooper on D-Day," Harold said. "I came down behind the German lines like all my buddies. I didn't know where

I was or where they were. It was pure terror. I saw all these terrible things, and I shot a lot of people. It's never out of my mind."

I immediately realized my cluelessness. I didn't know Harold well at all. Here was a true WWII hero trying to live a normal family life, trying to fight a serious illness, yet suffering from disabling post-traumatic stress disorder from fifty years past. Somehow, I hadn't found a way to listen deeply enough.

But Harold's defenses took hold again rapidly.

"I'm sorry, Doctor. Sometimes it just grabs me."

I tried to reach out and refer him for counseling, but Harold would have none of it. "Doc, it's OK. I don't want to see some shrink."

In future office visits he continued to deflect questions about PTSD, though Harold's wife confided that he had frequent night terrors, shouting in his sleep and awaking drenched with sweat.

Harold survived two more years until his pulmonary fibrosis finally caused his demise. I wish I could say that his death was peaceful, but as he weakened the terrors took hold and would not leave. Our palliative care team used enough sedation and narcotics to essentially put him in a medically induced coma. But Harold's PTSD didn't really die until he did.

THE LAKE WOBEGONE EFFECT

There are two very interesting books about how we, as doctors and patients, approach health care. One, *How Doctor's Think,* offers exactly what the title suggests: insight on how doctors tend to approach their work. The other, *Your Medical Mind,* helps patients understand the complexities of medical decision-making. My takeaway after reading both? Very often, we are at odds. The way "we" think and the way "they" think do rarely connect.

In the ICU, for example, I was often perplexed at the tendency of families to be unrealistically optimistic about the survival of their loved ones. I'd say that, statistically speaking, the patient had perhaps a five percent chance of survival—that is, a

95% likelihood of dying—and even less if the patient was on a ventilator with multiple organs failing. But the families, though they intellectually understood the notion of poor probability, still believed they would beat the odds, much like a gambler, I suppose, though with higher stakes.

Educators are familiar with the Lake Wobegone effect in that almost all parents feel that their children are above average. When it comes to health care in the ICU, a recent study[4] confirmed a similarly optimistic bias among the families of patients. It's natural, of course, when confronted with the possible loss of a loved one. It's our default to martial all available resources to keep them alive—including near-delusional optimism in the face of dire facts.

But it also offers a partial explanation for the difficulty physicians have in shifting from full-bore heroic ICU care toward palliative comfort. The standard in medicine, traditionally, is to keep going with life-prolonging measures. So this change is nothing less than existential for a doctor, suggesting that we think it's OK to die, which can cause profound moral distress for physicians and nurses, as well as families.

For this reason, physicians are reluctant to make statements like, "Your wife is dying and we are doing everything possible to make her comfortable, but I don't recommend CPR or heart shocks, which could cause pain and also be ineffective." But without this kind of clarity about the pros and cons of medical intervention, confusion reigns. And sometimes conversations are complicated. There may be trust issues between a family and physician. Or different cultural approaches to death and dying. If we, as doctors, understand that patients and families are generally biased toward optimism, we can, by listening with empathy, help them bridge the gap between their expectations and reality.

WHO'S IN CONTROL?

Discussion and shared decision-making around death require great sensitivity. At times, these talks become a tango between doctor and patient, even a battle for control. Vonnie, one of my early patients, taught me some important lessons about this. But first I had to learn to listen.

I was just starting out when Vonnie came in as a patient. She looked me in the eye and said, "I'm here because I have sarcoidosis. I've looked you up in the Directory of Medical Specialists, talked to friends who know your work, and I've decided that I want you to be my doctor."

I could see right away that Vonnie was a woman who liked to take control of whatever situation she confronted. And I quickly surmised that she might be challenging to care for. Vonnie taught medical terminology to medical assistants so she knew all about pulmonary functions, rales, wheezes, and every organ that could be affected by her disease. I tried to assert control or at least set boundaries. But I was still quite young, and with Vonnie, everything was a negotiation. We came to an agreement about which tests needed to be done. But treatment was another matter.

Sarcoidosis was named for its lumpy, red lesions and literally means "flesh-like." (The word *sarcasm* actually means "cutting through flesh"). These small clusters of lymphocytes can multiply and congregate in any organ of the body, most often the lymph nodes, lungs, liver, eyes, and skin. Researchers have spent decades searching for the cause—an infectious agent? Some kind of environmental exposure? Lots of theories have led up blind alleys. Thankfully, most patients with sarcoidosis have a benign course, often enjoying complete spontaneous resolution. But Vonnie's disease was serious. It had attacked her lungs, where it progressed relentlessly.

The most common course of treatment at the time was the steroid prednisone, which has significant side effects. Vonnie put up with the most benign ones—weight gain, puffiness, bruising. But the mental effects she found impossibly disabling. Vonnie complained of feeling spacey, irritable, just not herself. It had strained family her relationships, which were all-important.

"I just need to stop the prednisone," Vonnie told me.

I was very worried about this and pushed back hard.

"Vonnie, if you stop the prednisone your sarcoidosis will certainly worsen. It could shorten your life."

Vonnie did not seem to mind.

"That's OK," she said. "I'm so much happier without the side effects, come what may."

Over time, I learned to truly hear her and cede to what was most important to my patient. This was Vonnie's life and her choice about how to live it. She knew the options. Slowly, she tapered off the prednisone and felt healed.

"Dr. deMaine," Vonnie would ask, "you do remember Francis Peabody's dictum, don't you?"

I nodded: *the secret of the care of the patient is in caring for the patient.*

The Latin root for doctor, *docere* means "to teach." But in this instance, Vonnie taught me. The lesson was to elevate that which mattered most to her, mental health.

As Vonnie's condition worsened, her family rallied. She was a devout Catholic, and it helped her to persevere. "We Catholics understand suffering!" she would say with a laugh. The end came quickly, likely from a pulmonary embolism. Later, Vonnie's family told me about her wake. She'd had it all planned: the music, the poems, the silver, china, and crystal—and she'd directed that all would raise a glass (or two) and wish her well in her new adventure with God.

A few days after her death, a note arrived in my in-box: "Dear Doctor deMaine, because it is the aim of the physician to heal and to extend life, it must have been difficult for you to let go and allow me to reject the steroids. Yet without the anxiety produced by the prednisone, my spirit is healed. I am 'myself' again. I did not ask for a personal healing at Lourdes, only that the cause and cure of sarcoidosis be found. As a result, I am able to embrace life and to live it with a great degree of peace. My children now know me as I am and can learn that death is a companion, not a tyrant. In your own inimitable way, you've given me the kindest of care—a mirror of the love with which God tends me. Thanks, and prayers, Vonnie."

THE PHYSICAL EXAM—A LOST ART?

Sometimes nobody is listening well, or the patient's history is incomplete, and the path for effective treatment has been lost. Bobby, a thirty-seven-year-old farmer, was admitted to the hospital with overwhelming fatigue and shortness of breath. Yet he looked the picture of health. Bobby had grown up rising before dawn, milking cows, and working long days in the field. He had never been seriously ill as a child, and in high school played halfback on the football team.

But this was Bobby's third admission for evaluation. He had been through heart and lung tests and even a psychiatric examination, but everything was coming up normal. As is usual at a university hospital, the first doctor to see Bobby was a third-year medical student named Mike, who was himself being examined for his ability to evaluate patients.

Mike spent about an hour going through Bobby's extensive chart: normal blood count, electrolytes, liver function, kidney function, calcium, and thyroid tests. The urinalysis was normal, as were the chest x-ray and EKG. Bobby's condition had baffled the medical residents, research fellows, and faculty—so what in the world could Mike contribute as a lowly medical student?

Bobby told his story once again: "I feel OK when not doing much, but when I try to climb a ladder or haul some hay I just feel all-in. There's no pain, but I just feel like keeling over." A treadmill test confirmed this; Bobby's endurance was quite limited. But there was no sign of coronary artery disease.

Mike noted this and began again from scratch with a new evaluation. This included Bobby's chief complaint, followed by a description of the present illness, past medical history, family history, travel history, and social history.

"I'm going to ask you a bunch of questions you've probably been asked before, do you mind?" Mike asked.

"Not if you can fix me up. I don't want to die from this," Bobby said.

"OK, let's start all the way back. Tell me your story about growing up. I need to know all I can about you."

So Mike became a listener, and Bobby began to tell stories from his childhood, some of which we're pretty entertaining—like the time he tipped over an outhouse at Halloween, with a farmer inside!

"That guy was as mad as a hornet," Bobby continued. "In fact, we were running away, and when I climbed over a fence, he cut loose with his shotgun. Maybe he was just trying to scare us, but I took some buckshot in my rear."

This intrigued Mike. He hadn't found anything in the prior records about trauma. "So what happened?" he asked. "Did you need surgery?"

"No, but there was a bunch of skin holes, and we only got one or two pellets out. It looked like I had chickenpox on my ass!"

Mike tucked this bit of information away and finished up his interview. He knew it would take hours to write up the notes for his examiner. But as he listened, Mike could not stop thinking about the puzzle of Bobby's shortness of breath. It didn't seem to be heart disease, lung disease, or any other organ failure. So what was it?

On a whim, Mike asked Bobby if anyone had ever listened to his bottom with a stethoscope.

"Now wouldn't that be something! Nobody's touched my butt outside of my wife, that's for sure!"

"It probably sounds a little crazy, but I'd like to check you there to see if the buckshot caused an unusual injury."

"Hey, Doc I'm desperate. If you think putting your stethoscope on my ass is the answer, then what the heck," Bobby laughed.

With Bobby prone, Mike could see the buckshot scars across his right buttock and thigh. He didn't notice any pulsations, but when he placed his hand over the area he felt a gushing sensation—in medical terminology, a "thrill." There was a clear vibration with each heartbeat. Through the stethoscope, Mike heard a loud "murmur."

He wasn't sure if this was the problem or, if so, whether anything could be done to fix it. The next day, Mike knew, he would be questioned by his mentors about these findings. Students, residents, and faculty came to Bobby's bedside. He couldn't contain himself. "Hey, my bright young doctor here has found a murmur on my ass, how about that!"

Mike sighed. This wasn't how he'd planned to present the problem. He gave the gunshot history and detailed the physical findings. The junior staff were skeptical about its significance. But the senior cardiologist recognized the brilliance of Mike's discovery.

"It's pretty clear that this patient has high output heart failure," he said. "I would guess that he's losing 50% of his cardiac output to a shunt between a large pelvic artery and vein. He can function OK at rest, but goes into high output heart failure with exercise because of the shunt."

That turned out to be the case exactly. Bobby's shunt was viewed with a dye contrast study and the vascular surgeons consulted. A large artery and vein had been fused by the penetrating trauma of the buckshot. The operation to close this shut and return the blood flow to a normal pattern was relatively straightforward. And afterward, Bobby was on his way.

I wish I could say that I was Mike in this story. Instead, I was one of the many doctors who missed the diagnosis. But I did learn that many medical problems can be uncovered by obtaining a detailed medical history and following it with a solid physical exam. As one professor said, "Listen to the patient with your eyes, ears, hands, and stethoscope." These days, to the chagrin of many, physicians have moved away from taking a comprehensive history and physical in favor of check-box medicine focused more on measurements and data collection. The drivers are economic, naturally, but there are often hidden costs.

This a poem by Danielle Hope, first published in *JAMA*, offers a contrasting view about the power of touch.

The Laying on of Hands[5]:
Priests offered it in weekly benediction to bless
after chants and motets, in Eucharist
or Mass, to magnify a union or to heal
the sick. Doves were sometimes released.

Lovers do it too. The caress—careless or casual.
The home from work, the comfort me, or the moment
when hands become all scent and skin; the arch of wrist,
the smooth palm and pure white fingernail tip.

So doctors learned it, palpated sick limbs, gauged temperatures,
pulses; probed chests, abdomens and necks to fathom symptoms,
interrogate signs. But now machines seek better, deeper,
further, filling the walls with images, bright and cold.

VIVA PUERTO VALLARTA

Jerry sat by his mother's bed saying, "Mom, hurry up and get well so we can go to Puerto Vallarta. Hey, we'll have a beer there."

The problem was there was no way to tell if anything was registering with Midge Jackson, Jerry's mom. She was on life support, heavily sedated, and things did not look good. Jerry was a firefighter, often on call in nearby Bellevue. But every free moment he could spare, he was with his mom, and as her doctor in the ICU, I had frequent communication with him.

I'd first met Midge and her family in medical crisis—unfortunately, not an unusual mode of initial contact in the ICU. The call came from my surgical colleague. "We're sending a patient to the ICU post triple A, and her blood pressure is falling. Could you see her?" The "triple A" was an abdominal aortic aneurysm replacement in this seventy-six-year-old woman. The large trunk of an artery in her lower abdomen was threatening to burst, and she had just barely survived the urgent surgery that replaced the aneurysm with a sizable graft.

At first, Midge seemed to improve, and we thought she was stabilizing. But then intestinal bleeding began. Midge got blood transfusions. Then the GI specialists found stress ulcers in her stomach. They got the bleeding controlled, but she remained on life support. Midge's lungs began to fill with fluid. The ventilator wasn't providing enough support. We were concerned about giving too much oxygen or too little, too much pressure or too little ventilation. It was difficult, but I told Midge's family that she had a reasonable chance of pulling through this new complication, acute respiratory distress syndrome.

At week three in the ICU, Midge's lungs were barely better, but they weren't worse, either. Jerry, the firefighter, kept saying, "Come on Mom, get better. Remember, we're going to Mexico." Midge was minimally responsive, but she could open her eyes and move all her limbs, so the family knew she was still there.

At week five, after surviving a bout of urinary infection, Midge's temperature spiked to 104, and her blood pressure and urine output fell drastically. We did the usual cultures and big gun antibiotics but found that a fungus was now growing in her blood. Things looked grim. Some of the staff began to wonder if we were doing Midge any favors by keeping her alive this way. But Jerry pushed back, challenging us: "I don't think you can say she has a terminal diagnosis, right? Do you think she does?"

We were now at eight weeks. There were frequent family conferences. Some of Midge's relatives began to think along the same lines as the medical staff. They weren't sure that Midge would want to keep going like this. But all of them described her as a vital person who loved life and "wouldn't go easily."

I felt that the family was indeed acting in Midge's best interest, but I told them that if there were any further complications, like a stroke, heart attack, or kidney failure, the outlook would be bleak indeed.

One day in the tenth week, like magic, Midge's bowel function returned, her blood count normalized, and her lungs began to clear. We lightened sedation, she began to respond, and we started weaning trials off the ventilator. Jerry kept saying, "Mom remember, it's Puerto Vallarta for a cerveza."

After nearly three months in the ICU, we celebrated the day that Midge was able to transfer out to the medical unit. It felt like a graduation. But Midge's efforts at rehabilitation had only just begun. She needed lots of strengthening and physical therapy. At that point I lost track of her, though I heard that she'd gone to a skilled nursing facility for intensive physical therapy. Then, months later, I had a surprise.

In the spring of the year Midge was discharged from rehab, I was at Sea-Tac Airport with my wife and kids, waiting to board our flight to Mexico—Puerto Vallarta, as it happened. Out of nowhere, I heard a shriek from across the lobby. "There's my doctor! You saved my life!" All I could see was an elderly, white-haired lady, and I was startled to realize that she was directing her shouts at me. Then I saw Jerry, and it all came together. We were on the same flight to Puerto Vallarta, and once we'd arrived we met over a cerveza.

Midge's case was one that the nurses and I often discussed later—in part, because her recovery was so gratifying. But it was also among the most humbling experiences of my career. We had grown discouraged, wondering if it was wise to push on with life support. The huge advantage that Midge had on top of a non-terminal condition was her advocate, Jerry, who just kept pushing. We had many care conferences with him, talking about Midge's wishes. Every time, Jerry said, "keep going"—and he was right. I often felt that Midge, too, was listening.

CANCER? HOW MUCH TIME
WILL YOU GIVE ME?

Ben's first symptom was coughing up blood. But his cancer had been silently growing for months, if not years. He had no pain or shortness of breath. But a chest x-ray showed a large mass at the root of the left lung, and the subsequent CT scan showed enlarged lymph nodes, which meant that the disease had likely spread to Ben's liver.

"So Doc, what is it? Cancer? How much time do you give me?"

As a pulmonologist, I saw conditions like this once or twice a week, but usually when the patient was a smoker. Ben was not. At forty-nine, he'd been a basically healthy guy.

But I didn't know Ben well—this was our first visit—nor his family, or life situation. It was far too soon for me to guess about Ben's future. I needed to figure out what was going on first. The usual plan of action included blood tests, a CT scan, and a bronchoscopy to determine a diagnosis before making any pronouncements. But Ben pressed. "Come on, Doc, give me your educated guess."

"My crystal ball is cloudy and I can't read your future, but I promise I'll tell you all I know as we go along," I said.

Bronchoscopy (from a pulmonologist's point of view) is a relatively simple outpatient procedure. With a lidocaine spray to numb the vocal cords and a short-acting sedative, we pass a flexible scope through the nose into the airways, and all of it is visible on a video monitor. It's like viewing the inside of a hollow tree trunk with all of the major branches in view. Ben's tumor was evident in the left main stem bronchus—red, rough, angry-looking tissue. While he watched the monitor, we biopsied his tumor. I showed him the findings and explained that we would have a diagnosis the next day.

It was a non-small cell carcinoma of the lung—the most common type.

"OK, now how long do I have?" Ben asked.

Small lung cancers that are near the periphery of the lungs have the best outlook and are often curable. But Ben's cancer was Stage 3B.

How should I answer Ben's question? Where is any patient on the statistical curve? How can we begin to know what their response to treatment will be? In the last decade, we've seen significant improvement in treatment and survival rates among some lung cancer patients, but that often means a few more months of life, not years.

So this is how I answered: "I don't have the powers of a deity and can't see the future, but here are the broad statistics. I'm hoping you not only beat the averages but become an outlier. You're younger and healthier than many of the patients in these studies. And you're not a statistic. I'm sending you to the best cancer treatment and research center available, so let's see what they have to say. But it's going to be one day at a time. You have to hope for the best and prepare for the worst. I'd like to see you again once a plan is in place."

Giving a patient "time" can be self-fulfilling so doctors typically exercise great caution in these conversations. At the same time, refusing to lay out realistic outcomes based on statistics denies a patient information that they often want, and are entitled to know. Sometimes, patients want more certainty than we can ethically provide. But it's the human connection that makes medicine powerful and humane. And it's important not to dodge the issue of death. As we've seen, when patients reach the stage of dying, doctors often fail to step in and say it's time for hospice and comfort care. We need to get much more comfortable with mortality and frailty—both our own and our patients'.

MY HUSBAND DIDN'T WANT THIS

Howie was voted outstanding teacher by the pediatric residents year after year. He was a walking textbook on the classic diseases of childhood: measles, mumps, and whooping cough. Over lunch, he'd rail against the ways allergists tested kids. "Can you believe they tie them to a papoose board, inject all these allergens up and down their back, look for swelling and redness, and call it a positive test?" he'd cry. "Then they put the kids on dust and mold shots!"

Howie loved the science of medicine. But his greatest passion was patients. He had an amazing rapport with children. One mom reported that Howie would all but ignore her, in favor of hopping onto the exam table to blow up a balloon and start talking with her six-year-old. Kids loved going to see "Doctor Howie."

He retired ten years ahead of me, and we lost touch. Then one day I got a call from Howie's wife, Jeannie. He'd had a severe stroke and was in a nursing home. "I don't know what to do, and I really need some help," Jeannie said. "Howie keeps getting pneumonia. He's confused and can't move his right side. Could you visit him?"

I asked Jeannie how she was holding up.

"Not very well," she said. "I feel so badly for him. They put in this feeding tube, which I'm pretty sure he wouldn't have wanted. One thing just led to another during rehab, but he's not making any progress."

We chatted some more. As his spouse, Jeannie was Howie's advocate by default, now that he wasn't able to make his wishes known. He had not completed an advance directive.

Nursing homes are often called God's waiting room, and in a way that's accurate. Many residents exist in a sort of limbo state—out-of-sight, out-of-mind. When I went to visit Howie, he lay propped up in bed, his jaw slack, his right eye partly closed. He did not respond to my voice or hand squeeze. The nurses had been unable to rouse him. There wasn't much for physical therapy to do other than passive range of motion exercises.

I spoke with Howie's neurologist. The prognosis for meaningful recovery looked bleak. Again, Jeannie said, "I know he would hate being like this. But I'd feel so guilty if I had his tube feedings stopped. I don't even know if the facility would allow that."

We found a quiet place to talk. Howie and Jeannie's two grown sons joined us. Fortunately, all three were in agreement. Howie would never have wanted to live like this. Together, they developed a picture of what he would wish for, what he would say if he could, and how he would love them for listening. They talked with their minister, a close friend, a social worker, and their doctor. A week later, after the feeding tube had been removed, Howie died peacefully.

TOO YOUNG

Marcie, at nineteen, was far too young to die, which made it hard for all of us to face the impending reality. Her pediatrician had suspected the problem shortly after birth. Marcie wasn't growing normally, and she had more respiratory infections than most children. A sweat chloride test proved conclusive for cystic fibrosis (CF). The diagnosis was devastating to Marcie's mom and dad, both of whom were free of the disease but carriers of the gene for it. Statistically, this meant that 25% of their children would have both abnormal genes, and thus have CF. Marcie was the unlucky one.

Her mom, Sally, was committed to learning what could be done. But Marcie's dad, Rich, was angry about the whole thing and distanced himself. By the time Marcie transferred to my practice, Rich and Sally had divorced.

Sally, like many parents of CF children, had become well-versed in the care, advocacy, and support for kids with this disease. She'd learned that CF problems are related to thick mucus secretions in the lungs, and that a variety of aerosols could help. Early treatment of lung infections was important, as was constant monitoring of the fat-soluble vitamins in Marcie's blood (vitamins D, E, A, and K). In CF patients, the pancreas does not secrete enzymes normally so enzyme pills are often part of the daily regimen, along with vitamins.

Once or twice a year, Marcie had severe respiratory infections requiring hospitalization. The rest of the time, she was excelling in school and growing into a lovely young lady. She hoped to train as a nurse and, in her early high school years, volunteered at a local hospital. She had started dating and had a wide circle of friends.

During one of these hospitalizations, Marcie complained of "peeing all the time." I asked if anyone had checked her blood sugar. It turned out to be 310 (normal is less than 100). Her pancreas was failing, and she was now diabetic, further complicating care. Additionally, her liver was becoming involved, and she'd had some bleeding from veins in her lower esophagus, which required more intervention.

Despite all of this, Marcie tried to set goals for herself. Average lifespans of CF patients have increased dramatically. In 1938, their life expectancy was just six months. Today, a child born with CF can live to middle age. But Marcie, now nineteen, had so many complications and hospitalizations that her outlook was looking progressively worse. She knew her time was limited so her goals became very near-term.

This left me with the challenge of discussing end-of-life issues with a young woman about to graduate from high school. Marcie had seen other CF kids die, and she found discussing her own mortality deeply depressing. She indicated that if there was truly no hope, she wouldn't want to keep going on machines.

All along, Sally had encouraged her daughter to "go for it" and live life. And as Marcie neared the end of her senior year, she set her heart on going to the senior prom. She considered it an all-important, once-in-a-lifetime event. She knew it was risky, health-wise, especially as the deterioration of her lungs had continued, so as the day approached she and her mother had a heart to heart. Sally truly didn't want her daughter to go to the prom. She was terrified of losing Marcie and already grieving the loss to come.

"Mom, I've got to go," Marcie pleaded. "It's once in a lifetime!"

You can imagine how Sally struggled. She knew it was dangerous, but she also knew that Marcie's time was short. Despite the health risks, her daughter's happiness mattered more. Marcie, delighted, went out for her big night and had a wonderful time.

Within a week she suffered acute respiratory failure. With Marcie gasping and blue, her mother called 911. Marcie was intubated at home, taken to an emergency room, and placed on a ventilator. She came under my care in the ICU, but there was no improvement. Marcie required heavy sedation to keep from pulling out her tubes.

Her mom and I had daily conferences. Sally was reluctant to accept that her daughter was not going to get better, and she resisted thinking about the end. I discussed the situation with a colleague who had treated Marcie previously and had good rapport with her family. He told Sally that he agreed with my assessment: Marcie would not survive off the ventilator. Keeping her alive this way was only prolonging the dying process.

In the end, Sally and I agreed that before removing any tubes, we would wait until Marcie's nineteenth birthday, which fell the next day, a Saturday. On Sunday, Sally, Marcie's sister, boyfriend, and pastor assembled at her bedside. I turned off all the monitors in the room and gave them time to say their goodbyes. Then I asked the family to step outside. The nurses and I gave Marcie enough sedation for comfort, removed her endotracheal tube, and brought the family back in. They held her and talked to her until the very end.

"When she was a little girl, I dreamed of so many things for Marcie," Sally said to me through tears. "She was stronger than I was, and she helped me through my sadness. And she did achieve her goal—going to the prom."

Sally had been able, despite her terrible sadness and fear, to listen to this brave young woman about what mattered most to her.

ONE MORE TRIP TO GUAM

Marie was also too young to have a terminal diagnosis. She had primary pulmonary hypertension. This condition is called "primary" because we have no idea of the cause. Medical lingo has a variety of ways to label unknown causes, such as "idiopathic" or "essential." In Marie's case, the word was "primary," though none of these labels convey any level of deeper understanding. In any event, primary pulmonary hypertension is a devastating diagnosis that affects adult women about three times more often than men.

Marie was a soft-spoken woman of Asian descent, who had been born in Guam but lived in the U.S. for many years. She'd raised three children and helped her husband's business as a bookkeeper. She had a beautiful smile and tended to downplay her symptoms. Her family physician had referred her to me for puzzling shortness of breath.

A non-smoker who had been healthy all her life, Marie's lung function was normal, but she had some swelling of her ankles. Her heart tones were normal except for a split-second sound, a sign of delayed closure of the pulmonic valve, which leads from the heart to the lungs. The EKG showed strain in her right ventricle. All of this pointed to possible pulmonary hypertension, which was later confirmed by heart catheterization and cardiac ultrasound.

We ruled out causes like fen-phen or blood clots and began drug treatment to try to dilate the vessels going to her lungs. Essentially, all blood returning to the heart from the rest of the body needs to be pumped out to the lungs, where it gives off carbon dioxide and picks up oxygen. It's normally a low-pressure system, but not in Marie's case.

Over the next few years she began to fail. We tried other drugs and even a battery powered continuous IV medication, in addition to oxygen treatment. In the midst of all this, Marie decided to make her annual trip to Guam, where many of her relatives still lived.

I wanted to make sure she was stable enough to travel, so I reached out.

"Marie, how are you doing?"

"Oh, fine, Doctor. A little limited, but I can't complain."

I asked her to come in. Upon examination, it was clear that her condition had grown much worse. Marie was short of breath, her oxygen levels were lower, and her legs more swollen. We needed to consider more drastic measures.

"Marie, your condition is becoming life-threatening. The drugs are not working, and your cardiac echo is showing very high pulmonary artery pressure. I'd like to refer you to the university hospital to consider the possibility of a lung transplant."

"Oh, I'd never want anything like that."

"Why not?"

"I'm at peace with God," Marie said. "What will be, will be. I don't expect miracles, and surgery seems so risky to me. I think I'd rather just go on."

I asked Marie to bring in her husband, Gerald. He was seldom in the exam room with her, and I wanted to make sure he understood the seriousness of Marie's situation. She smiled at him when I brought up lung transplantation. Gerald smiled back.

"Look, Doctor, we've already talked about this," Gerald said. "Marie doesn't want surgery. She knows her time is short, and we're flying back to Guam next week. We'll be there a month."

I began to understand something important. Marie and her husband were further along in accepting impending death than I was. As Catholics of strong faith, they had a kind of fatalism that I didn't often see in my practice. They had accepted Marie's fate, while I was still ready to fight on.

I OK'd her for oxygen use on the airline. Marie arranged for additional oxygen in Guam. During the month she was there, I received a postcard saying, "Don't worry, I'm OK."

But upon her return to Seattle, Marie was much worse. She had episodes of severe shortness of breath, could no longer walk across a room, and was becoming bed-bound. Marie and Gerald agreed to a hospice referral.

From that point on I received regular updates from the hospice nurses, who were keeping Marie comfortable with small doses of morphine. After a few months of home care, the hospice nurse called.

"Doctor deMaine, we're wondering if you could visit Marie at home. She and the family would like to see you."

I didn't know what to expect when I left the office at 6 pm to stop by their home in a pleasant, suburban neighborhood. A child shyly answered the door and called for her grandpa, Gerald. Inside, the scene was surprisingly festive. Large dishes of food crowded the dining room table. There was music on and kids running, playing. In the middle of it all lay Marie in her hospital bed, her head propped up so she could see all the activity. A sleepy smile crossed her face as I walked into the room.

"Why don't you get something to eat, Doctor, you must be tired and hungry."

I sat with her for a while, listened to her chest with my stethoscope, and held her hand. The warmth and love surrounding Marie and her family were palpable. I felt tremendous respect for her emotional strength in facing death.

Within a week, Marie was gone from this life. But she'd left behind a beautiful legacy of love and acceptance. This was a blessing for her family and for me too—a healing.

I came away moved and inspired, hoping that I could someday face my own death with such equanimity, and that when it happened, I would have my loved ones close by. Marie's family had listened to her, and they were able to give her wonderfully caring support.

A word here about caregivers. Marie had a cadre of people tending to her, which allowed her to live out her last days as she wished, at home. But not everyone has this kind of family. Hospice provides caregivers with training and support, but frequently, the needs of family caregivers get overlooked. There are caregiver parents with disabled children; seventy-year-old women caring for ninety-five-year-old parents; young wives caring for husbands who have been injured or paralyzed—and so many more. It is estimated that fifty million people in our country are serving as caregivers, unheralded and unpaid. They too need support before, during, and after the death of a loved one. Often, they suffer in silence.

WHEN IT DOESN'T MAKE SENSE

I've always found medicine humbling. There's far more knowledge available than we can absorb, and it continues to expand exponentially. As doctors in training, we are taught to think in patterns, using "clinical judgement" to match a patient's presenting symptoms to a diagnosis. This works okay—until we are presented with an unfamiliar pattern. We may listen, but we don't know the right questions to ask.

In the early 1980s I saw a sixty-year-old shoe salesman with fatigue and a low-grade fever—an FUO (fever of unknown origin). He had general malaise and some muscle weakness. His exam and initial blood work were unremarkable except he was mildly anemic and his sedimentation rate (the rate that red blood cells settle in a tube of blood) was elevated. A search for cancer and infection showed nothing notable. My next thought was polymyalgia rheumatica, an autoimmune illness associated with arterial inflammation. I ordered a temporal artery biopsy, which was negative.

About this time, my patient developed a cough, and his chest x-ray showed a hazy pattern of change. I had read about this strange new medical problem, but had only seen one patient with AIDS. It was not established in my pattern of thinking. My patient turned out to be one of the first cases in Washington state, but we had likely missed many others. Clinically speaking, pattern thinking usually works. But it isn't a good way to ferret out anything new or unexpected.

In this case, for example, I'd never thought to ask the right questions. So I missed the fact that my patient was gay and never suspected HIV. I was too complacent, in other words. I thought I'd covered my bases for all the many diseases that can cause an FUO—a list of nearly one hundred illnesses. But we don't know what we don't think of. My patient went on to contract full-blown AIDS and died as most patients did in the early days of the HIV epidemic, before we'd developed the effective therapies that exist now.

Another time, a young man with shaking chills and fever was referred to my clinic. I immediately suspected viral or bacterial infection and tried to narrow down the possible causes. But the patient made my diagnosis for me, "Hey, Doc, you know I felt just like this when I had malaria in Vietnam."

It was dramatic to see the parasites in his red blood cells when I went to the lab. But again, I felt humbled to have missed this by focusing on the familiar patterns and standard shortcuts we tend to use in everyday medicine.

Patients are endlessly varying in their presentations, and there are still so many unknowns—Covid-19 being only the most recent example. One of the most important lessons I learned in medical school is something I ponder daily: "The questions in medicine never change, but every few years the answers do."

Some of the best primary care physicians I know seem to have a sixth sense when a patient's story and exam don't add up. One day a GP friend called me for a phone consult. "Jim, I've got a patient here who was diagnosed with pneumonia in Europe. She's home now, and I don't think she should be this short of breath. She can't even handle a flight of stairs. She's never been limited like this in the past."

As a pulmonologist, I immediately thought about air travel and blood clots. My GP friend, looking at his patient through a different lens, hadn't recognized that pattern. He just knew that things didn't sound right. It turned out the patient had survived a major pulmonary embolus and still had dangerous clots in her legs. She started on anticoagulation treatment, and it cleared up the problem.

When I was a medical resident at a VA Hospital, we had a long-term patient with a knee joint infection. He had been there for a month with a staph infection, which had now turned into an even more difficult pseudomonas infection requiring fairly toxic IV medications, plus knee joint drainage. As that knee slowly resolved, the other knee joint became septic. This just didn't make sense. My intern sent the patient downstairs for x-rays and then checked the bedside table. Sure enough, there was a vial of cloudy, infected urine along with a collection of syringes and needles that the patient had been using to self-inject his knees. The rare diagnosis of Munchausen's Syndrome was our answer. Munchausen's is a psychiatric disorder in which patients induce a variety of medical and surgical illnesses in themselves or others who are close to them.

These varying situations taught me not only to listen, but to question my assumptions. We have to be suspicious of what's out there that we don't know. It's constantly humbling. Medical learning only starts in medical school. But it never stops.

CONFLICTS

E n route to becoming a doctor all medical students learn the eth-ical principle, "First, do no Harm." But who decides how that mandate is interpreted? When a physician offers a procedure or treat-ment, what are the potential benefits—and what are the potential harms? Patients have the right to know, in order to make an educated decision about what is the best course of action for themselves. This is the basis of "informed consent." But at times, even with good medical practice, things don't turn out well. Sometimes no error is involved but sometimes there is. How should doctors deal with mistakes? Can we ever say we're sorry?

YOU KILLED MY MOTHER

Martha's death was difficult but not unexpected. She had been in and out of the hospital three times in the past six weeks. Her severe COPD had finally caught up with her. Intensive medical treatment was failing, and she did not want to be placed on a ven-tilator. Her husband was there at the end.

The next day I got a call from their son, John, who lived locally but hadn't been around much.

"Doctor, you killed my mother!" he shouted into the phone. "I want to meet with you and my lawyer—today!"

I was not particularly worried. John had not been part of his mother's treatment. He never showed up for her appointments, or called to talk about her prognosis. Martha and her husband had prepared for the end. Yet John seemed shocked by it. Perhaps he was estranged from them, or unaware of how ill his mother had been. I really didn't know. But I was confident that Martha had been well cared for.

I'd just had a patient cancel, so there was an unexpected opening in my schedule.

"Sure," I told John. "How about 2PM?" I think it surprised him.

I arranged for us to meet in a conference room since I didn't know how many people would be there. Medically, I didn't think I had done anything wrong, so I decided to try handling the situation myself. I was fairly certain that if I alerted the hospital's legal department they would want to talk with me first and then attend the meeting. But I had been through enough contentious situations over the years to realize how that might escalate tensions.

I ordered up all of Martha's records and brought them to the third-floor conference room next to the library. Four of Martha's family members arrived: John, her son; Ed, her husband; Paul, her brother-in-law, and Sue, her sister.

Was their lawyer coming? I asked, a bit perplexed. Paul answered he was a tax attorney. Apparently, this was whom John had meant when he'd threatened to bring his lawyer.

After introductions, I asked John to explain his concerns regarding his mother's care.

"I think she got too much morphine, and it killed her," he said.

I let them know that I wished things had turned out differently, and that this was a sad loss for the family. But "sorry" is a tricky word in such circumstances. It can imply a mistake, and none had been made in this case. Martha's COPD had simply stopped responding to treatment.

"Let's review the care and medications she received," I said. "First, I think we all understand that Martha had very severe emphysema, and she was eighty-one years old. She was getting weaker as her lung function worsened, even though we were using prednisone and inhalers. She also had lots of infections, which we treated with antibiotics. But she was slowly suffocating, even with oxygen."

"Well, where does the morphine come in?" John said.

"Good question. Martha let us know that she didn't want to be put on a ventilator because her quality of life was so poor. But it made her panicky when she couldn't catch her breath. She said it felt like she was drowning. Indeed, her carbon dioxide levels were climbing and her oxygen levels falling. The end wasn't far away—"

"OK, but what about the morphine?" John interjected.

"Well, your mom was becoming agitated. She was crying out, not making sense. At that point, I talked to your dad and told him morphine or a sedative would help your mom be more comfortable. So we put her on small doses to titrate care for comfort, and to relieve her shortness of breath."

"Is that right, Dad?" John said, turning to his father.

"Yes. Mom was so uncomfortable and so confused. We needed to do something to make her more peaceful. I felt that she was dying."

I could sense John softening, as he listened to his father and began, slowly, to understand.

"Let's look at the medication sheet," I said. "The nurses gave your mom 1 or 2 mg of morphine at each of these times over a three-hour period. The total dose was 10 mg. Although it's possible that the morphine hastened her death by a few minutes, it did several very positive things for her. It relieved her anxiety and decreased her sense of drowning. Basically, it relaxed her enough to drift into sleep and, ultimately, death. Without the morphine, she would have had a miserable end."

By now John had calmed down and begun to realize that he needed to support his dad. And I'd learned an important lesson: all family members need to be involved at the end, with active outreach if they can't be present. The mistake I'd made with Martha's family was lack of communication. Over the years, I would come to insist that every member of a patient's immediate family take part in end-of-life conferences.

Nowadays, with technology, that is much easier to facilitate. But still, when navigating the stress of a terminal condition, it is easily overlooked—to everyone's disadvantage. Allowing all concerns to be aired and addressed, with transparency and a frank admission of any shortcomings, is a better way to go. In this case, I should have brought John in much earlier so he could understand the palliative use of morphine in end-stage lung disease. I learned the hard way that there's a direct correlation between distance from care and anger after the fact. When family members feel don't feel included, they are likely to be hurt. And often, that hurt morphs into anger.

BRAIN DEAD

Sam was late, and Ella was furious. "Why isn't that man back by now? He knows it's time to leave for church!"

Hours passed, and Ella became frightened. Sam had gone out for his usual two-mile run and simply disappeared. Ella called friends and neighbors, but no one had seen him. Ella began to panic. She called 911, which connected her to the police.

"No ma'am, we've had no reports with anyone by that name."

In desperation, Ella began to check area hospitals, but they also had no knowledge of Sam. Ella checked in the bedroom and found his wallet, car keys, and cell phone. "Of course they don't know anything about anyone by that name," she realized. "He has no ID on him."

Finally, she got through to an administrator with the medic crew. That morning at 10:03 a.m. they had received a call from a Metro bus driver that a man was down on the sidewalk and not moving. The Medics found him not breathing, with no pulse, and his heart in ventricular fibrillation. CPR and shocks got his circulation reestablished, and he was admitted to the trauma center as a "John Doe," kept on life support. When Ella arrived at the hospital and found her husband in the ICU, she reeled. A tube protruded from Sam's mouth, another tube was in his nose, a heart monitor was quietly beeping, and IVs flowed into his neck and arms.

"Is this really happening? Have I lost him?" Ella thought to herself, while trying to be brave for her two teenagers. The family was in shock.

Sam had gone into cardiac arrest while jogging, and his heart rhythm had come to a standstill. Now his heart, lungs, and kidney were all working again. But what about his brain?

Over the next few days Sam underwent extensive testing. There was no significant brain activity visible on an EEG. Even more discouraging was the complete lack of blood flow to the higher centers of the brain. Sam's body did not even attempt to breathe when the ventilator was paused for a brain death protocol. Any hope of Sam returning to his prior life was nil. He was legally dead.

The criteria for brain death are quite stringent. The Uniform Determination of Death Act (UDDA), enacted in 1981, defines it this way:[1]

An individual who has sustained either (1) irreversible cessation of circulatory and respiratory functions, or (2) irreversible cessation of all functions of the entire brain, including the brain stem, is dead.

So a person may be declared brain dead even as their heart and circulation continue. This is not any kind of coma; legally, the person is dead. But explaining that to a family can be difficult. Their loved one does not look dead. But they are, even if circulation is ongoing.

Sam became my patient and my responsibility when he was transferred to my hospital's ICU for "ongoing care." As a treating physician, my obligation is first to the patient and then to the family. Sometimes this is easy, but sometimes loaded with conflict. Fortunately, Sam and Ella had a strong family with two beautiful teenagers, Adella and Isaiah, who wanted to help their mom.

Together, we discussed the hopeless situation of Sam's brain and the options of continuing ventilator support (a better term here than life support since, legally, he was no longer alive), along with a feeding tube. A staff neurologist explained the total absence of meaningful brain function. The family met with their pastor, then with a hospital social worker. They felt that Sam would want to be removed from the ventilator and allowed to die naturally, peacefully.

When I went into the ICU that afternoon, I listened to their pastor reading to them from the Bible: *"For as the rain comes down, and the snow from heaven, and returns not thither, but waters the earth, and makes it bring forth and bud, that it may give seed to the sower, and bread to the eater. So shall my word be that goes forth out of my mouth: it shall not return unto me void, but it shall accomplish that which I please, and it shall prosper in the thing whereto I sent it. For ye shall go out with joy, and be led forth with peace: the mountains and the hills shall break forth before you into singing, and all the trees of the field shall clap their hands."*

They were celebrating Sam's life, it seemed to me. And the pastor further explained, "The soul is present, but the body too damaged to further clothe the soul. The real Sam will live on."

Yet his body, while on life support, was still functioning. His organs were still alive. Ella and her children were quite taken aback when a transplant coordinator asked to meet with them. The ICU staff, per protocol, had notified the regional transplant center about a potential organ donor. Ethically, it was important for me to keep my distance from the transplant team and remain focused on Sam, my patient. So Ella, the kids, and their pastor agreed met with the transplant coordinator to discuss how Sam might benefit others as a donor—possibly more than a dozen people. Through saving their lives with his organs, he could in a sense live on.

But the prospect made Ella queasy. "Isn't this disrespectful to him?" she said. "How can I allow my husband to be cut open when he's barely dead?"

As with most medical innovation, the ability to perform transplants has opened a whole new arena of ethical questions. In 2016, a patient with ALS on a ventilator said he wanted to donate his organs by being admitted to the hospital and removed from breathing support. His doctors agreed but hospital attorneys felt this was too close to assisted suicide. The ALS patient was denied.[2]

In Sam's case, there was no such confusion. He was gone, Ella prayed, and in the end said she found greater peace by carrying out Sam's wishes to be a donor. The children appeared bewildered, but they accepted this decision. Their tears flowed.

Although Sam had never completed any advance directives, he had done the most important thing. He and Ella had had that all-important discussion about their hopes, fears, and what mattered most to them in life. Sam had told her, "I would never want to be a vegetable. If that happens, let me pass."

As Sam's spouse, Ella was legally his surrogate. In this regard, he had done her a huge favor by letting Ella know his deepest wishes about life and where he drew the limit.

I'm not sure how many organs were harvested from Sam. His heart was allowed to stop for one hundred and twenty seconds to ensure that death was complete (no heart will spontaneously restart after that time period), though he'd been legally brain dead for three days already.

There will likely be continued debate about what actually constitutes death. Although brain cells choked of oxygen begin to die off within five minutes, some can be retrieved and grown in a laboratory for hours after death. So when is a person truly dead?

Eight years after Sam's passing, I received a phone call out of the blue from Ella.

"Hi, Dr. deMaine, do you remember me?"

Some patients stand out, and I immediately recalled the trauma of Sam's death. Ella said she wanted to thank me for my care, but she was really calling to let me know that the children had both graduated from college. Then, shyly, she mentioned one more thing.

"For the first time since Sam's passing, I've started a relationship, and am so happy!" she said, noting that while the pain had never completely disappeared, life had presented her with an unexpected new chapter.

WHO GETS THE ORGANS?

Transplants are not always such a peaceful experience, however. I recall sitting in a meeting with a pediatric surgeon who looked utterly miserable. I had no idea why.

"Is anything wrong?" I asked.

"I just came from harvesting the organs of a twelve-year-old boy killed in a bike accident, and I can't help thinking about my own kids," he said. "It was so hard. I just tried to keep thinking about all the good these organs could do."

As technology advances, we are faced with ethical challenges that were unimaginable in the past—not least, how to decide who gets treatment when resources are scarce. These kinds of questions started coming to the fore in 1962, when a new era in lifesaving began with the first outpatient kidney dialysis clinic. It was founded in Seattle by Dr. Belding Scribner, and spurred a wellspring of demand for this new form of treatment. But at first there were few facilities that could provide it. Ethics Committees—labeled "God squads" by medical students—were set up to wrestle with these questions and make the call: who should get treatment, and who, by default, would not?

The concept of organ transplantation had been around since 1954, when Joseph Murray transplanted a kidney from one identical twin into another. But the procedure didn't become mainstream until years later with introduction of the anti-rejection drug cyclosporine. Once again, innovation would create an entirely new problem: long lists of people now waiting for donor kidneys, hearts, lungs, and livers. My friend Dan was among them.

"How come my ankles are so swollen? I can barely get my shoes on," Dan said to me one day. We were on a trip together with our wives, far from medical care, so I suggested that it might be varicose veins or an overly sedentary lifestyle. "When we get home, try some support stockings," I suggested.

In the back of my mind, I was a little worried about blood clots. But I never even considered kidney failure. Several weeks later, after he'd had a series of blood tests, Dan called me.

"Jim, my numbers are off the chart. I have only about 17% of kidney function left."

Dan's doctors couldn't pinpoint the cause of his shrunken kidneys. But they had been failing for years—perhaps since childhood. Medications and an altered diet did nothing to slow the decline. Dan was seventy-two-years-old at this point. Realistically, what were the options?

Staff at the kidney center felt he was a bit old for a transplant. But if the rest of his health was excellent, he might qualify. To ensure this, Dan underwent multiple prostate biopsies to rule out cancer; he had a heart catheterization, lung testing, and a full body CT scan. All looked fine, so Dan was entered onto the list of eighty thousand people waiting for kidney transplants in the U.S. About a third of them would die before receiving one.

Meanwhile, Dan began peritoneal dialysis at home. It was a new and uncomfortable reality. He might be dying, but maybe not. Living in limbo affected his sleep. Each day, while a gift, brought new challenges. His solid family bonds—a wife, two children, and five grandchildren—gave Dan the strength to keep going, and his faith was a comfort as he pondered death. But the waiting was a huge emotional drain.

Dan heard that he could get a transplant immediately if he flew to India, an option he rejected after learning that destitute people there are sometimes paid to sell their organs for such procedures. The medical concerns were secondary for Dan. A transplant like that would be simply immoral, he felt.

Two friends offered to be live donors. This floored Dan. Would he have done the same? Neither friend turned out to be a match, so Dan's wait continued. One night after about fourteen months of this, he got a phone call. Be ready, said the doctor on the other end. There is a possible donor. Dan and his wife waited for hours to hear more—only to learn that the donor's organ was in such poor shape that it was unacceptable for transplant.

The wait continued, but Dan was getting discouraged. His legs were growing numb, despite vitamin therapy, and the emotional drain was wearing on him. But finally, the call came and Dan was off to the hospital.

"A kidney is coming from somewhere, and I may never find out where or who. I'm just so grateful that they've given me a chance!" he told me over the phone.

The operation went well, and Dan was back home in a few days. That did not mean he was out of the woods, however. Viruses attacked, as they often do after transplants, and it took nearly six weeks on fairly toxic drugs before Dan felt healthy.

Not long afterward, the organ donation team got in touch and asked if Dan would like to write an anonymous letter to his donor's family, explaining what their gift had meant to him. He wanted to do this, but found it difficult to express the depth of his gratitude.

By then, the two of us had signed up to be volunteer advocates for organ transplantation, and we were invited to an appreciation dinner. I am the recipient of two partial corneal transplants, so it was personal for me as well as Dan. At our table that night sat a heart transplant recipient and his wife, as well as a thirty-eight-year-old computer programmer from Microsoft who had just undergone surgery as an anonymous kidney donor. "Why not?" he'd thought. He had no idea who the recipient might be, but someday, he said, he hoped they would meet.

Dan could hardly get the words out. "You know, I'm a kidney transplant recipient," he said. "It's a great thing you've done."

SEEING THROUGH ANOTHER'S EYES

Like Dan, I have tried to write a letter of thanks to the family of the person whose gift saved my sight. But it is unexpectedly difficult. I don't know what to say or even how to begin. I don't know the persons I am writing to, but part of their loved one is literally now a part of me.

I never anticipated someday becoming an organ recipient, and though my situation was not life-threatening like Dan's, it was life-changing.

The journey began with a phone call from my brother. "Jim, what the hell is Fuchs' Dystrophy anyway—do you have it too?"

My brother's vision was growing hazy, and he could no longer track the flight of a golf ball, or even a baseball hit with a hard line-drive. He couldn't read clearly until early afternoon. The problem was that his cornea (the outer layer of the eye) was waterlogged. Blowing a hairdryer into his eyes helped some, as did a strong solution of salt water. But these weren't real answers, and the problem was worsening.

An ophthalmologist explained that this was an inherited disease. We knew our parents' eyesight wasn't great. But both of them had passed away by the time my brother called me, and neither had ever been diagnosed with Fuchs'. The treatment options were three: no treatment (which would lead to scarring and blindness); a traditional corneal transplant; or the relatively new Descemet's membrane transplant called DSAEK, which is essentially a partial corneal transplant.

The cornea, I discovered, is an amazing part of the body. This window for sight has five layers and, with its curvature, provides two-thirds of the refraction needed for clear vision. The innermost layer, the endothelium, produces a membrane that pumps water out of the cornea to keep it crystalline clear. It's our very own sump pump, built into the cornea. In Fuchs', the endothelial cells start to die off prematurely. As a consequence, the cornea starts to swell, affecting vision.

My brother chose to undergo the DSAEK procedure in both eyes and had stunning results. He's now back to golf (without a spotter) and has excellent vision.

But then it was my turn. Initially, I thought the problem was cataracts. But it turned out that I was, like my brother, unlucky in the inheritance chain. The transplant procedure took place in my own clinic, where I knew everyone. But to maintain the appropriate professional demeanor, they asked my name and birth date three times, for safety controls, just like they would for any other patient. I'll admit it, this all felt quite strange. I was sedated, but conscious, as the surgeon made a tiny incision, stripping a button of the ineffective endothelium from my eye and replacing it with a similar-sized button from a cadaver. A few months later, I did the same with the other eye.

The willingness of people to donate their corneas, along with the advent of eye banks and dramatic advances in corneal surgery are now benefiting thousands of people.

But what about the donors? I hadn't given them much thought until I tried to write my letter of thanks. My transplant was minor, compared with the stakes involved in a kidney or lung transplant, yet every time I open my eyes I know that everything I see comes by the grace of this thoughtful person, unknown to me, who wanted to give part of themselves to others.

I have so many questions. What happened to my donor? How old was he or she? Was their death expected or sudden? How can I fully express all that I feel—gratitude hardly seems to cover it. I've always checked the organ donor box on my driver's license and never actually thought what that might mean to someone else. But the fact is, as I write these words I am seeing them through someone else's eyes.

THE OBECALP EFFECT

I've spent a good part of my career puzzling through medical ethics. These can be high-stakes conundrums, or everyday riddles—such when doctors administer placebo treatments. Is it ever OK to bend truth-telling in an effort to improve the quality of a patient's life? The ethical principle of beneficence sometimes clashes with autonomy—a patient's right to make their own choices. I have rarely been asked to prescribe placebos, but there was one instance I remember well.

Betty's complaints were escalating. She'd been living in a nursing home for four years and wasn't happy. Every month she came up with new symptoms: aching, fatigue, nervous stomach, tingling, and dizziness among them. In response, her daughter, Nancy, took Betty to the doctor for endless diagnostic tests: blood counts, liver functions, x-rays, thyroid function, and many others. Everything came back normal. Betty's neurologist and rheumatologist had been unable to find anything wrong. And though Betty

was getting a bit forgetful, she wanted to be in charge of everything—her finances, health decisions, and daily life.

Nancy didn't know what to do. Her mother was demanding
and increasingly unreasonable. All she seemed to want was more
medication. But nothing soothed her symptoms. "Honey, they just
aren't doing anything for me—nothing at all," she'd complain.
"I'm not sleeping. I ache all over. Something's got to be done!"

Nancy and I served on a board together, and she asked if I
would see her mom in consultation, just to review things. I met
with Betty in my office. She was well-groomed, talkative and controlling. "Doctor, you just have to do something. I'm suffering
and no one pays any attention. I think they're all a bunch of idiots,
don't you?"

She was also pretty sharp. Betty loved to talk politics, and she
could reason quite well. Her tests showed no cancer, inflammatory
illness, or metabolic problems. In other words, I couldn't come up
with anything, either.

"Can't you just give her a placebo?" Nancy pleaded, when I
broke the news.

This was a number of years ago, and our clinic pharmacy carried a "drug" called obecalp. As you may have gleaned, this is "placebo" spelled backward. I had never prescribed obecalp, but it was
doled out now and then. Nancy begged me to try it on her mom.

"Why not?" she said. "I know doctors don't want to deceive
patients, but it can't do any harm. And I'm desperate. So is my
mom!"

The placebo effect is real, though not well understood. It
exemplifies the mysteries of the mind-body connection in human
health, and we are not sure why it works about a third of the time
for real pain. The word itself comes from Latin, meaning "I shall
please," and technically, prescribing a placebo is prescribing hope.
For some patients, that seems to do the trick.

Under today's rules about transparency and patient autonomy
in the U.S., this would be considered unethical. But a survey of
nearly seven hundred internists and rheumatologists published

in the *British Medical Journal*,[3] found that about half said they prescribed placebos on a regular basis. Several years ago, Harvard University even created an institute, the Program in Placebo Studies and the Therapeutic Encounter, wholly dedicated to the study of the placebo effect—including the question of whether placebos should become part of standard medical practice.[4]

Even if placebos are officially frowned upon, many supplements, diet aids, cold remedies, cough medications, and antibiotics are given without convincing evidence that they are useful or necessary. Alternative medicine also capitalizes on beliefs and rituals that appear to have healing powers which are little understood. No less a figure than Sir William Osler, one of the founders of modern medicine, said, "The desire to take medicine is perhaps the greatest feature which distinguishes man from animals."[5]

With more than a little reluctance, I gave Betty some obecalp for her plethora of symptoms. A few weeks later I got a call.

"You're not going to believe this," Nancy said. "Mom loves her obecalp. All is well."

It appears that a combination of laying on of hands, belief, a daughter's love, and the placebo effect all played a part in making Betty comfortable. She died in her sleep a few years later.

HONOR THE ADVANCE DIRECTIVE—OR NOT?

I gave a lunchtime talk at a retirement home to a group of about sixty highly educated folks, aimed at educating families about the value of advance planning and how to make their values and wishes known. The talk "Your Life, Your Choices" is one I give frequently, and my audience on this day included judges, chaplains, and professors all engaged in dynamic discussion.

As usual, I spoke about the value of advance directives for preserving patients' autonomy in decision making when they can no longer competent to speak for themselves. Afterward, a woman quietly approached and asked if she could have a moment of my time.

"My husband has worsening Alzheimer's and can no longer care for himself," she said. "He's been transferred to a Memory Care Unit. The doctors say he is no longer competent to make any health care or financial decisions, so the burden is entirely on me. But I have a problem. A few years ago, my husband said that he would want full life support, including fluid and nutrition tubes to sustain him, and he signed the papers saying so. But I don't know if that's the right thing to do now."

I asked if she thought CPR would benefit her husband if his heart stopped.

"No," she replied. "But I'm not certain what his wishes would be in that situation. He never talked about quality of life issues much."

This is kind of situation is why I advise people to write an addendum to their Living Will—while they are still competent—giving a personal interpretation of that term, "quality of life." Without such statements, it can be difficult for surrogates to make decisions on behalf of patients who are too ill to discuss their status. It's rarely easy in these gray-zone situations, and dementia directives[6] are being developed. In the meantime, a statement about your biggest hopes and biggest fears can go a long way toward helping. What is an acceptable quality of life for you, personally, and what would lead you to think it's time to "pull the plug"? The more we can let surrogates know our deepest feelings on these matters, the better their decisions on our behalf.

I tried to reassure the woman before me that doctors feel obligated to "do no harm," and that many would not offer CPR and intubation for her husband. I advised her to talk with his doctor and a palliative care or hospice provider, as well as a hospital social worker or spiritual counselor.

But she'd raised an interesting point, which I later discussed with a health care lawyer: what if your advocate's best judgement runs counter to your directive? In cases of advanced dementia, for example, you essentially become a different person from the one who signed that form.

The lawyer felt that this woman, as her husband's legal advocate, had leeway to interpret his wishes using "substituted judgement." If done in good faith, she was not necessarily bound by the letter of the document. In other words, circumstances can change, and rigidity in the face of new facts serves no one.

"Sometimes common sense outweighs the living will," the lawyer told me. "Yes, someone could sue that the letter of the document wasn't followed. But it's unlikely. Either way, the advocate has quite a burden to bear."

The point is that we all need someone with us at the end who knows our heart. For example, the composer Chopin, had one great fear about death: the possibility of being buried while still alive. According to Stephen Lagerberg is his book, *Chopin's Heart,* the musician was so adamant about avoiding this fate that he had his physician promise to remove his heart at death, thus ensuring that he was in fact dead! Chopin is buried in France, but his heart is enshrined in a church in Poland.

May we all have physicians that know our hearts and honor our wishes to this degree.

TALKING TO GOD?

Often, the ethics around patient autonomy conflict with the judgement of physicians and nurses earned through years of experience. But the concepts of beneficence and doing no harm are enshrined in the Hippocratic Oath. This tension brings up all kinds of difficult scenarios, like the following:

"We have a patient on a ventilator who is stable enough to transfer to your ICU, if that's OK." I was on call and about to become the attending physician for a critically ill woman.

Eighty-nine-year-old Stella Norris was incapacitated from a massive stroke she'd suffered five years earlier. She had a feeding tube inserted through her stomach wall and needed total body care. At home, her step-grandson, George, ministered to her. He had called 911 when she stopped breathing. The medics intubated her and brought Stella to the closest hospital.

This hospital had kept Stella longer than necessary, due to insurance issues between competing health care systems. But things went awry, and suddenly Stella's transfer to my ICU was deemed urgent.

The precipitating event, I learned later, was this: George was discovered in the ICU, disconnecting the endotracheal tube from Stella's ventilator and inserting herbal medications down the tube into her lungs. Alarms went off, and the nurses were so horrified that they hastened to designate Stella for transfer out of there. Yes, it would mean a loss of income for the hospital, but that was outweighed by getting a problem patient out of their hair.

I admitted Stella, and examined this debilitated ill woman. Her limbs were shrunken on the distorted right side of her body, and she did not respond to any verbal or physical stimuli. She had bed sores, infected urine, and a dense pneumonia that showed up in a chest x-ray. Her family said she has not been responsive or out of bed for five years. With some trepidation, I arranged a care conference with them.

Stela's adult daughter, Janice, seldom visited her mother because there is no ability to communicate. Home care had been given over to George, who devoted his life to tending Stella, day and night in his small apartment. George believed in miracles, he said, and spent his days reading about alternative therapies and watching televangelists on TV. He said that God spoke to him.

At our family conference, I asked about Stella's wishes for invasive care. Her daughter said there were no known advance directives.

"I'm really not sure mom would have wanted any of this," Janice began. "I'm certain I wouldn't want anything like this kind of extended care for myself, but...."

She trailed off, confused.

I explained Stella's poor outlook, and the way we were prolonging her death with the ventilator, tube feeding, and antibiotics. But there was a dynamic in the room that I couldn't figure out. George sat quietly with a scowl on his face, never nodding in agreement, nor voicing any protest.

"George, what are your thoughts?" I asked.

"I know she's not ready to die. God has spoken to me, and I know."

Janice and the other family members backed off. They didn't want to attend any more conferences, and deferred to George on all matters. He had been Stella's caregiver, after all, and they seemed reluctant—maybe intimidated—to challenge him, though I'd pointed out that he might not be acting in Stella's best interest.

The next week George posted a notice for Stella's memorial service in the ICU. He was predicting that she would die more than three months hence! It was chilling, to say the least. I brought the case to our Ethics Committee, and they asked the hospital chaplain to talk with George and the family. That failed too. The chaplain was unable to connect with George in any rational manner. Under Washington state law, Stella's daughter had legal decision-making authority, which we pointed out. But Janice again deferred to George. We contacted the hospital's legal department—maybe a court-appointed guardian could help? That route looked dicey, too, as few guardians were likely to countermand Janice's deference to George.

After eight weeks in the ICU, Stella's circulation began to fail, and her entire left arm was gangrenous. Our orthopedic surgeon refused to offer amputation because Stella wouldn't survive the surgery.

Around this time, I finally told George that I would be unwilling to do CPR or electric shocks to restart Stella's heart whenever it stopped. He gave me a vacant look. The nurses begin to worry about what George would do when his step-grandmother finally died.

But the end was unexpectedly peaceful. Stella passed away with George present. Her heart flat-lined, as the ventilator continued to puff fruitlessly. I received a call at home that evening.

"We need you to come in here and pronounce Stella dead. Otherwise, George might freak out," said the nurse on the other end of the line. "We don't know what this crazy guy might do! We need a doctor here. God has to speak."

I was exhausted and did not want to drive back to the hospital. But I needed an experienced, forceful physician at the bedside. I called a burly colleague who was in-house that evening.

"Don, can you do me a huge favor?"

After asking the nurses to alert security and have them present in the ICU, Don agreed to pronounce Stella dead and tell George. He received the news, left the hospital, and we never heard from the family again.

In some countries doctors have more leeway, and families defer to a physician on decisions about when to withdraw life support. The U.S. norm, however, is transparency, shared decision making, and an effort to work toward consensus. The problem in Stella's situation was that her wishes were never truly known, and the care was futile. Obviously, this raises the question of unnecessary use (and expense) of scarce resources like ventilators. If I were to manage Stella's case again, I would have involved our legal department sooner. Likely, they would have agreed that Stella's care was futile and given the family a few weeks to find another institution—which is not much of a solution, either.

WHY DO SO MANY BLACK AMERICANS AVOID ADVANCE DIRECTIVES?

I was speaking at a senior center in Seattle's Central Area, traditionally the hub of Black life in this city, attempting to talk about end-of-life planning.

"How can I be sure that a white doctor will believe me when I say I have real pain?" a woman in the audience asked. Others nodded around her. The audience wasn't hostile, just honest. Their experiences with health care had not predisposed them toward trusting white physicians.[7] In a discussion about making final wishes known, they doubted that anyone would really listen.

The audience was dotted with people who remembered the Tuskegee Syphilis Experiment, and others who recalled segregated hospital wards. One man, well into his nineties, told me about serving during World War II, subjected to Jim Crow laws as a Tuskegee Airman. "I wasn't allowed to eat, sleep, or socialize in any of the more elegant white areas, even though I was an officer," he said. Some eighty years later, the memory remained raw.

That same disparity persists today—most dramatically evident in the ways COVID-19 has devastated minority communities. Between service jobs that more commonly put people of color into contact with the public; a prevalence of underlying health conditions like hypertension, diabetes, and kidney disease which are themselves a reflection of longstanding social and economic disparities; and bias in health care access, Black Americans account for the bulk of Covid-19 fatalities.

Under these circumstances, advance care planning is more critical than ever—for people of every ethnic group.

Yet our health care system is far behind the curve in dealing with cultural diversity. In the face of daily discrimination, building trust is difficult. So many people of color avoid end-of-life preparation—including hospice.

"Many of us feel that hospice workers will take our dying loved one off to some institution where they won't have the comfort of us caring for them," one woman explained. "We are family-based, and we turn to God for help."

As a Caucasian, I'd often sensed this skepticism from Black patients, a hesitancy in answering my questions. Considering the history of systemic racism in this country, who can blame them? But now, here I was, talking about one of the most intimate decisions in any person's life: their death. Was I even qualified to speak to this community?

I was concerned enough to seek guidance from the Mayor's Council on African-American Elders, which is how I met Brenda

Charles-Edwards, the council's dynamic chairwoman. Brenda has trained to facilitate small groups in preparing advance directives in her community. She understood the importance of the information I wanted to impart, as well as the awkwardness of my being its messenger. So we began doing these talks together.

"Why are so few Black people completing advance directives?" I asked her during a radio interview between the two of us.

"For some, it's just too hard a subject, so it gets put off," she said. "They feel that if they talk about it and make plans, this will somehow make death come sooner. Others believe they won't be listened to—no matter what." (So why bother, was the meaning implied.)

The depth of distrust was not news to me, but I had not realized how deeply it permeated Black Americans' view of our health care system.

When giving these talks, I often show a video called, *Unequal Treatment*, about the widespread lack of trust in hospice within the Black community. In it, a pastor and his wife are navigating the tragic loss of two sons, both from sickle cell anemia. The first son's death had been excruciating, endured without any thought of hospice or palliative care. By the time the couple's second son faced the same illness, the pastor and his wife were working with a Black physician and, at his urging, reluctantly agreed to involve hospice so their son could get some relief. He died peacefully, in the arms of his family. A healing experience so profound that it affected the pastor's entire congregation.

Brenda works with families and small groups, modeling ways to hold these difficult conversations within a community that has long avoided them.

One time, we spoke at a forum for Black caregivers, and I gained a profound appreciation for the depth of sacrifice that is standard within this community. Routinely, Black caregivers will minister to a parent with dementia at home—even if it causes them financial or physical hardship. They are not interested in hastening death, viewing it as a process of passing from this world to the next that needs to happen on its own timetable.

SAFETY, RISK, AND COMPROMISE

At ninety-three, Alice knew she was a source of worry for her sons, but she refused to leave her beautiful family home on the shores of Lake Washington. She loved her privacy, and was willing to pay for part-time help with shopping and gardening.

Alice also knew that her heart's aortic valve was very narrow. She had put off surgery to get a new valve for fifteen years. And one day, she went into sudden, acute pulmonary edema, with blood backing up into her lungs which causing severe shortness of breath. Thankfully, a neighbor was visiting at the time and rushed Alice to the ER, where she was stabilized. But upon discharge from the hospital, Alice's doctors met with her three sons and laid out the facts: the same scenario might recur at any moment. Plans needed to be made.

Seniors often tell me that they want independence in their later years. They want to be able to take that long dreamed-of trip, or attend that wedding, or stay in their own home—even if it means risking a fall. They don't want to be governed by fear.

It reminds me of *The 100-Year-Old Man Who Climbed Out the Window and Disappeared*, a book by Jonas Jonasson. The hero of this story leaves his nursing home for an amazing adventure, rather than sit there celebrating his centennial birthday.

Alice was a bit like that adventurous character, quite clear that she did not want CPR, heart shocks, or a ventilator. "Boys, I've lived a long life, and am ready to kick the bucket when my number's up," she told her sons. "I don't want any bells and whistles. Just TLC."

I've heard much the same from geriatricians. Doctors who care for the aging focus on dementia, depression, fall prevention, over medication, and the complexity of interacting health problems. Nursing home administrators often list safety first. But nursing home residents don't. What they want is doctors who support what matters most to them—even if it compromises their safety a bit.

Alice's sons urged her to take a breath and think through her choices. They reviewed her Living Will, confirming her choice for no heroic measures. One was appointed her durable power of attorney for health, with the other two as alternates. But how would any of this help prevent an emergency?

"Let's look at the options," one son said. "You need more care, so come live with one of us. Or maybe we can hire a live-in caregiver."

Alice would hear none of it.

"Listen, this is my life, and I get to choose what I want," she said.

What to do with this impasse? How could Alice's twelve grandchildren, fifteen great grandchildren, sons and daughters-in-law honor her wishes for autonomy while making sure she'd be safe?

Alice's kids met with her physician and a social worker to come up with a plan: Alice and her doctor would complete a POLST form, specifying no heroic measures, and Alice wore a bracelet affirming her DNR status. The family then contacted their closest Fire Department stationhouse and spoke with its medics. Alice would start wearing a "panic button" around her neck to summon emergency care if necessary; the Fire Department would keep a copy of her POLST on file; and Alice would have a lock box on her door allowing medics to enter without breaking in.

For good measure, a copy of Alice's POLST went to her doctor and the closest ER. Several other copies were filed around her house.

"Now quit worrying—I may live forever!" Alice said with a smile. Her family continued to check on her twice a day, though she never saw the point of all that fuss.

SAILING TO HAWAII

I've never really understood tobacco addiction, how it seems to become part of who you are as it captures your soul. I once had a colleague, Steve, who was a beloved Chief of OB-GYN in the hospital where I worked and, unfortunately, a two-pack-a-day smoker since college.

He knew it was probably killing him, and he was also an avid sailor, so he tried to trick himself into quitting.

"Jim, I'm going to kick the habit this time," he told me. "I'm sailing to Hawaii and back—without cigarettes."

I didn't believe he could do it. He used to smoke in his office with the door shut—in violation of our clinic's no-smoking policy—until we set up a temporary smoking room. Sometimes, during a lengthy surgery, he'd leave midway through to have a smoke. Yet when Steve sailed off to Hawaii with his wife, Dorothy, he quit! He didn't smoke for two months.

But upon his return, it was as if Steve had never stopped at all. He said he couldn't feel normal without his nicotine fix. That is the power of addiction. He knew it would likely kill him. He'd tried nicotine gum and patches, hypnosis and acupuncture. Nothing helped.

At seventy-four, Steve's habit finally caught up with him in the form of advanced COPD. He could no longer walk more than a block and needed a portable oxygen system, along with prednisone, inhalers, and antibiotics. Every few months he wound up in the ER. Dorothy, a strong-willed woman, was utterly beside herself. Exhausted after years of nagging Steve, she began heading off, solo, on "trips of lifetime" just to clear her head. But she dearly loved her husband and always accompanied him on office visits.

After several hospitalizations, Steve was preparing for the end. He let me know that he did not ever want to be put on life support with a ventilator, nor did he want CPR. He had discussed these wishes with Dorothy, and though she did not necessarily agree with his plans, she promised to honor them as Steve's designated health care agent.

"Whatever he wants, I'll support him," Dorothy said.

The problem arose when Steve was admitted to the hospital once again, when I was out of town. A young colleague of mine, an excellent pulmonologist, evaluated him, and the conversation did not go well.

"Your breathing problem is critical. I'd like to move you to the ICU," my colleague said.

"No," Steve whispered, "I'm not going there. I don't want a ventilator!"

"Why not?"

"Look, just treat my shortness of breath and make me comfortable," Steve gasped.

Then Dorothy took the reins.

"Doctor, Steve really does not want life support. We've talked about it."

"Well, I think you both should rethink that. With a ventilator we could save his life."

The back and forth continued, with my colleague pushing for the ICU until Dorothy had finally had enough.

"Doctor, you aren't listening," she said. "Please leave."

Steve's wife had all the qualities we want in an advocate: she was a good listener, unafraid to stand up for her husband's rights, and undaunted in her support for Steve's wishes, even though they were not her own. I wish she hadn't had to push so hard, but sometimes that's what it takes. Steve died a few days later.

When families and medical caregivers can't arrive at a plan through shared decision making, it usually means that someone isn't listening. Fortunately, Steve had Dorothy to speak for him until the end. I heard from the nurses that she all but threw my colleague out of the room!

Later, he and I spoke about the confrontation. As a young doctor he hadn't yet come to the point where he was comfortable letting go. I walked him through this idea of respecting patients' autonomy, even when we might want to push on. I think he listened.

THE UNASKED QUESTION

Throughout the scenarios recounted in this book, there runs a common thread: the ethical questions that frame virtually every decision one makes in medicine, especially around handling mistakes.

A large, heavy package arrived at my office. I'd been expecting these medical records after my recent conversation with the attorney who'd sent them. He said, "Doctor deMaine, I'm representing a teaching hospital in a medical malpractice case related to a firefighter's death." He wanted me to review the records in hopes that I would testify as an expert witness. The hospital was being sued for failing to diagnose the massive pulmonary emboli (blood clots) that had caused the firefighter's death, and I was being asked to help defend the doctors.

The cardboard box contained hundreds of Xeroxed pages—autopsy reports of the patient, records from the doctors who had treated her, and further reports from doctors outside the hospital. I lugged all this home and spent hours that evening sifting and sorting the timeline of events.

It was a tragic story. This thirty-four-year-old female firefighter had begun to notice that she became easily winded during exercise. She saw her internist, who checked her heart and lungs, including a chest x-ray and EKG. Her heart rate was 90—higher than her usual 70, but within normal range and not enough to raise any red flags. There was no diagnosis for her symptoms. She saw this physician once more, which resulted in similar findings and a normal screening breathing test. Yet the discomfort during exercise persisted.

Subsequently, at a house fire, this young woman collapsed while attempting to scale a ladder, carrying a heavy hose, and had a brief seizure-like episode. Medics responded and she was taken to the hospital emergency department. Her blood pressure was fine, her heart rate was 110, and her neurological exam was normal. The neurology service admitted her for observation and a "seizure workup."

After two days in the hospital, there was still no diagnosis. The firefighter's shortness of breath history was noted, but her pulse never dropped below 110 (a red flag). She was discharged with an appointment to visit the pulmonary clinic in two weeks. Three days later, she collapsed at home in the shower. Her roommate called 911. This time, finally, she was diagnosed with a massive pulmonary embolus. But it was too late. In the x-ray department she had a sudden cardiac arrest and died undergoing CPR.

I combed through her outpatient history, looking for clues. I noticed, buried in her chart, that she had been taking birth control pills for the past six months. There was no history of asthma, allergies, or lung disease.

The attorney was not happy when I told him that I couldn't testify for the defense. It seemed to me that the doctors in the ER and on the neurology service had missed the obvious clues. They didn't note the history of birth control pills and ignored her rapid heart rate and shortness of breath. They were too focused on the "seizure-like episode" brought on by heavy exertion at the fire.

"Settle this one and try to stay away from a jury," was the best advice I could give.

"Look," I said, "if you present this case with the appropriate information, any emergency physician—even a medical student— would diagnose pulmonary emboli. You have a young woman on birth control pills who is becoming short of breath with a rapid pulse even at rest. This is a clear signal of possible blood clots clogging the lungs."

I explained that these clots, which start in the upper legs and pelvis, often have no local symptoms, but they can be deadly as they break loose and travel to the lungs. They impede blood flow and the circulatory system collapses. The "seizure" was a red herring. This woman never should have been discharged without a diagnosis. And why had they made her wait two weeks for a pulmonary consult when it easily could have been done during her admission? No one had put two and two together in this case. No one asked the right questions, so the correct diagnosis went unconsidered. A simple lung scan would have made this clear, and anti-coagulation would have saved her life.

The attorney told me I was being unhelpful to the medical profession, and angrily reminded me that I was prohibited from testifying for the plaintiff—the firefighter's family—which was certainly OK with me.

This was a very sad and preventable death. There aren't many things that cause a young woman on birth control pills to have severe shortness of breath, and a pulmonary embolism should have been among the first things considered. But because she was mistakenly believed to have had a "seizure," the firefighter was admitted to neurology. As I've noted in previous examples, each medical specialty tends to view patients through its own lens, looking for recognizable patterns. The smartest doctors have a sixth sense in cases like this, an ability to step back and ask the right questions. Fortunately, most of the time they get it right.

A FATAL TOOTH EXTRACTION

Though I didn't testify in the firefighter case, I have been deposed in other medical malpractice actions, and it's never a pleasant experience. In this one I was a treating physician, but not one of those being sued.

Don's wisdom tooth was acting up again. At age twenty-seven, he'd been fighting off recurrent pain, gum infections, and crowding of his teeth. Finally, his dentist told him it was time to see an oral surgeon. After x-rays, the oral surgeon advised Don to have all four wisdom teeth pulled in one sitting. The procedure was carried out a few weeks later. Don began taking penicillin tablets a day ahead, and the extractions went smoothly, except for one impacted lower tooth that was tough to remove.

The following day Don's jaw was swollen, as he'd anticipated. He had a low-grade fever and took some Tylenol. But on the third day, a Saturday, he wasn't doing well at all. His jaw was more swollen, and he was having trouble swallowing. He saw an on-call oral surgeon, who examined him and doubled his dose of penicillin. Another on-call oral surgeon saw him briefly on Sunday. By Monday, a holiday, Don was beginning to drool, and his voice was squeaky. Plus, his fever was 102 degrees. A third oral surgeon saw him and removed the stitches, switched antibiotics, and told him to see his regular oral surgeon the next day.

On Tuesday, as the admitting critical care doctor, I got a call from the ER.

"Jim, I've got a patient here brought in by the medics. He saw his oral surgeon today about chest pains and breathing problems, and their office called 911 because of a possible heart attack. He has some bizarre findings. Can you see him right away?"

In the ER, it was obvious that Don was critically ill. His breathing was painful and shallow; his voice high pitched and squeaky. He was perspiring, with a temperature of 104, and had a racing pulse of 130. The nurses were busy getting blood cultures, blood gases, starting an IV, and retrieving his chest x-ray.

I was startled when I felt his neck and upper chest. There was a crackling feel, medically what we call crepitus, which signifies air in the tissues. Had Don's lung collapsed? His tongue was so swollen and protruding, I couldn't see the back of his throat. His lungs showed diffuse abnormal crackles, and even his heart had a rubbing, crunching sound. A chest x-ray indicated air shadows in the soft tissues of the neck, shoulders, and chest, where no air should be. There were also large collections of fluid around both lungs. But because there was no evidence of a collapsed lung, the air could only be from gas-forming bacteria growing there.

We admitted Don to the ICU where he was seen by both otolaryngology and thoracic surgeons. His breathing was so marginal that he required a ventilator. His neck and chest had to be opened surgically and drained. Then we performed a tracheotomy. The foul-smelling gas came from three species of bacteria common to the mouth, plus a few others.

Over the next twenty-four hours Don seemed to rally, but he had further complications of bleeding, dense pneumonia, and heart arrhythmias. In seventy-two hours, he was dead, leaving behind his devastated wife and child.

Ludwig's angina was described by Wilhelm Frederick von Ludwig (1790-1865). This critical emergency is fairly rare these days with early detection and antibiotics, but Don's case was a classic example. The problem was the delay in recognizing the severity of the infection and the critical importance of early intervention. Getting sick on the Friday of a holiday weekend was unlucky timing. Seeing four different oral surgeons on successive days did not help. Each had passed the buck, hoping Don would get better without their doing much, and all failed to respond adequately to his distress.

The kind of wide drainage required in Don's operation is especially difficult. But in this case, delay of diagnosis and treatment were the critical failures.

As a treating physician, I was deposed when the case became a lawsuit. My understanding is that the oral surgeons' partnership broke apart, and they settled for the maximum under their insurance policy—small recompense for Don's loved ones. Is there anything else Don or his family could have done? There was no reason for them to have thought an immediate trip to the ER was warranted. And Don had followed-up day after day with the oral surgeons on call. It is quite likely none of them had ever seen Ludwig's angina before, as it is quite rare. And as it was a holiday weekend, each oral surgeon was covering for a colleague—none really giving in-depth opinions. This resulted in fractured continuity of care. These are not excuses, just factors in understanding Don's case. When mistakes happen, several things need to line up wrong.

SORRY SEEMS TO BE THE HARDEST WORD

No field is immune to error, including medicine. But many mistakes turn out to be of little consequence; our bodies are resilient and can fend off many assaults of nature. Similarly, a patient can receive a wrong medicine and never know it. But breakdowns in communication can be disastrous. When doctors are involved in a situation that goes wrong, can we say the hardest word?

There was a test we used to perform in the 1960s, in which a solution was injected intravenously to measure a patient's liver metabolism. The vials were stored in a basket at the nurse's station for us to use as needed. Nestled in the same basket were vials of epinephrine, used for severe allergic reactions. The vials looked similar and, regrettably, a fourth-year student in the class above mine injected a large dose of epinephrine IV into his patient.

"Oh, my God, my head!" the patient gasped, as his blood pres-sure soared. Then his heart stopped and could not be revived. I don't know if there was legal action afterward. But I do know that the epinephrine vials were quickly moved to a locked cabinet and labeled differently.

Another time, I learned about a fellow intern who needed to push fluids aggressively into a very ill patient. In those days, we had glass IV bottles instead of the plastic we use now, which are easy to compress with a blood pressure cuff if necessary. The intern, without thinking it through, decided to pump air into the glass IV bottle to speed up the delivery of the IV fluid.

It worked. But when the intern turned his back for a moment the bottle ran dry, and a large amount of air was pumped into the patient's circulatory system, obstructing blood flow through the heart, which caused his death. This physician eventually left clinical medicine for a career in research.

A patient in the ICU was diagnosed with recurrent lymphoma. The oncologist called in an order for cytoxan, prednisone, and vincristine. But the recorder on the other end of the line, who was working a double shift, mistakenly wrote a prescription to take the vincristine daily for five days, similar to the prednisone. Vincristine should be given only on day one. Over the next four days, the patient absorbed a fatal dosage and died of bone marrow failure. In this case, however, the oncologist apologized to the family in person, the hospital carried out a mortality review, and oversight systems were refined. Now, all medication orders had to be reviewed and signed by an oncologist before initiating. Training for pharmacists and nurses was updated. There was no lawsuit.

I saw a similar result when a radiology department doctor accidentally injected cleaning solution—rather than dye—into a patient's femoral artery, leading to a painful death. The vials of clear fluid had been placed close to each other on a procedure tray. Hospital representatives met promptly with the family, apologized for the mistake, and offered a financial settlement which was eventually accepted. Again, procedures were reviewed and strengthened to prevent similar accidents.

As a doctor, it's devastating to be involved in a serious mistake. I recall sitting down with a psychiatrist friend after I'd made a significant error, and it helped to talk it out. But the hospital's legal department had to be notified, affected family members faced, and reports made to the state (all of this in the middle of a sixty-hour work week). Fortunately, I was not sued, but the worry was crushing. My fatal mistake occurred during a procedure that I probably shouldn't have attempted because the patient was so sick. I sat down with the family afterward and explained the whole sequence. The man's son peppered me with questions. But then he paused, reflected, and said, "It must be hard to be a doctor sometimes. Look, it's OK. Dad was going nowhere, and he's in a better place now." Basically, he let me off the hook.

Most medical errors are the result of stress and fatigue. How best to deal with all the parties affected—the patient, family, providers, institution, legal department, and insurer? The answer is simple but simultaneously difficult: apologize![8] Mistakes can be honestly dealt with. In many states, a doctor's initial discussion with a patient's family about a mistake is not discoverable in a lawsuit. This promotes transparency, and data shows that, from a legal standpoint, 'fessing up[9] is the best thing to do. Certainly, from the moral point of view that's true. But when you're humiliated and ashamed, it's not so easy to confront your failings.

An apology is best made face-to-face. Phone calls and letters are second choice. Email is not effective at all. Sometimes a doctor or medical team is forgiven, sometimes not. But an honest, unqualified admission of error is the best way to release pressure, cool a family's understandable anger, and come to some sort of settlement for making amends.

A true apology should have the following elements:

- Say "I'm sorry." Not "I'm sorry but ..."
- Own up to the mistake, and admit you were wrong. The person must know you are accepting responsibility for the damage you've caused.
- Describe what happened. This may help clarify misunderstandings.
- Outline a plan to help make things better.
- Humbly ask for forgiveness.

Things to avoid in an apology:

- Justifying your actions.
- Saying "I'm sorry you were hurt by my words/actions" but not admitting they were wrong.
- Pushing back on the feelings of the other person.
- Going off-point and talking about other things.

It's hard to stay angry at punish someone who looks you in the eye, actively listens to all of your concerns, and sincerely apologizes. There comes a point that we recognize that we're all only human.

I'M SORRY I HAVE TO SUE YOU

I felt sad when I went to make rounds in the hospital. One of my patients, a colleague, had been readmitted in poor condition for recurrence of a primary lung sarcoma. I spent a few minutes examining Dennis and we chatted. He looked at me strangely in a way I didn't understand until he said, "Jim, I know I'm dying. My wife and kids are still pretty young. I'm going to have to sue you.

"It's nothing personal," he added, noting my shock. "I know you've given me good care. But my wife is upset, and she blames you for where I'm at now. I don't have much life insurance or any other money for them to live on, so I guess the hospital and others will be named too."

There wasn't much more for me to say.

"Dennis, I can find another attending for you if you'd like."

"No, I want to stay with you."

Dennis was a well-liked family doctor. About five years earlier a "coin lesion" had been discovered on his chest x-ray. This 2 cm spot in the right upper lobe of the lung had a smooth, rounded border and didn't contain calcium. A CT scan showed no enlarged lymph nodes and no other spots. We biopsied the lesion but couldn't diagnose his condition. All we knew was that this abnormality was new. An x-ray five years earlier had looked completely normal.

In surgery, Dennis's right upper lobe was removed, along with local lymph nodes. The lesion turned out to be a primary lung sarcoma, an unusual type of cancer. One of the lymph nodes was also positive. We sent Dennis to local experts on sarcoma, and he got opinions from several cancer specialists. Consensus at the time was that sarcomas don't respond well to either chemo or radiation therapy. But after collecting a few more opinions, Dennis underwent a series of radiation treatments.

After that, we waited. For three years, there was little change. Dennis's cancer neither improved nor worsened. But then fluid began to accumulate in his right lung cavity, and the area where he was getting radiation saw some increased density. (Not a good sign.) I drained the fluid from Dennis' chest several times, but found no cancer cells. After more signs—but no proof—that the cancer might be progressing, I sent Dennis to a top chest surgeon who attempted a complete removal of Dennis's right lung in order to try to eradicate the entire residual tumor. The post-op was stormy. Dennis required ICU care with a ventilator for almost three months. And the sarcoma was never completely obliterated. It kept growing in Dennis's lymph nodes and the lining of his chest wall.

When Dennis was finally transferred back to my hospital and he told me he was going to sue, I met with his wife, Alice, who'd focused a year's worth of anger over her husband's tragic illness and suffering on me. It was awkward, to say the least, for me to remain involved, knowing a legal threat loomed.

I felt Dennis's care had been good so I wasn't terribly concerned about being challenged on that. But it usually takes several things to go wrong before someone brings a medical malpractice claim: a poor outcome, communication breakdown, anger, and a mistake or oversight of consequence. I wondered what I could have done differently to handle the situation better. To this day, I'm still not sure.

Toward the end, hospice met with Dennis and Alice and mercifully provided palliative care. Alice balked at the idea of having hospice at home. So Dennis died peacefully in a hospital hospice unit a few weeks later.

I later learned that Alice had tried to find an attorney to file suit, but that several experts, after reviewing Dennis's records, advised her that she had no grounds legally to forge ahead with a complaint. Sometimes even with good medical practice, the outcome is tragic.

TRIAL OF A CARDIOLOGIST

I went to court recently and sat quietly in the gallery, listening to the testimony of two experts who criticized a cardiologist's care. The case at first glance didn't look very good for this defendant. The patient had presented to the E.R. with atypical chest pain. He was admitted and evaluated with an EKG, cardiac enzymes, an exercise test, and nuclear medicine heart scanning. The results were all within normal range and he was discharged to follow up with his primary care physician, but told to notify the cardiologist if he had any further chest pains. He died of a massive heart attack four months later.

The two plaintiff experts questioned the cardiologist's interpretation of the tests as normal, and said that the care did not meet accepted standards. They both felt that the patient should have had a coronary angiogram to rule out narrowing of the coronary artery. The patient's autopsy, they noted, showed narrowing of two major coronary arteries, which had been the cause of death.

The defendant cardiologist was about forty, well trained and admired in local circles for his brilliance and excellent patient care. He was experienced in interventional cardiology—doing heart caths, stents, and angioplasty. He'd elected not to do an angiogram based on established national guidelines. Also, importantly, neither the patient nor his primary care doctor contacted the cardiologist after discharge from the hospital. Over the intervening four months, the man's chest pain had recurred intermittently, but he never told the cardiologist about this worrisome symptom. His primary care physician knew about it but referred him, mistakenly, to a gastroenterologist.

The first expert quibbled about minor EKG findings and the quality of the stress test, among other things. But his reasoning was circular and, to me, unconvincing. Although he was board certified and a member of the clinical cardiology faculty at a prestigious medical school, he'd never actually done a coronary angiogram.

The second expert had been flown in from the East Coast. He had Ivy League credentials, but had never trained in invasive cardiac procedures like coronary arteriography. On cross examination, this expert admitted that his bills for the case totaled more than $11,000, not including fees for his most recent consultations and the flight to testify in Washington. He had testified in multiple lawsuits across thirty-five states, almost always for the plaintiff.

Both experts, in other words, were guns for hire, willing to travel anywhere for a paycheck.

I later asked one of the attorneys how they identified and con-tracted medical experts to testify against doctors. "Oh, that's no problem," he said. "There are web sites that list all kinds of experts for these kinds of cases."

They don't come cheap. After adjournment for the day, I asked one attorney about the fees for bringing in expert witnesses. She said it was a career for some of them. "I know of a chiropractor who brings in more than $500,000 a year by testifying," she told me. "It's common to charge $400 to $500 an hour, but some ask up to $1,200, and they expect to be paid in advance!"

It's not always easy to find doctors willing to testify against other doctors. We've all made mistakes so who are we to point a finger? For that reason, finding experts from outside the area is common—but three thousand miles away, as our second expert was, felt extreme to me. He must have been accumulating plenty of frequent flyer points.

Aside from the hourly fees, flying in experts for depositions gets expensive, so a case must be worth at least $250,000 before most attorneys will even consider going ahead with a lawsuit. With their 40% contingency fees, these attorneys might net $100,000, and they're spending much of that upfront, just paying for their costs. So they hope for the home run case, like a wrongful death, to clear more than $1 million after expenses.

I certainly felt sorry for the deceased man's wife and adult chil-dren. But must someone always be to blame? Sure, lots of patients might have had coronary angiographies in this situation, but is that because it's legitimately indicated, or is it for other reasons like financial incentives? Our cardiologist could have charged a nice fee for that procedure, but he'd followed his best judgment and used accepted guidelines.

I sat there, pondering malpractice litigation and wondering why we ask a jury of lay people to sort out difficult medical quandaries. In this case, the jury was attentive. They asked probing questions when given the opportunity. But I wondered how they felt about these "hired gun" experts. I wished I could hear their deliberations.

In medical malpractice cases like this one, are there ever really winners? A man was dead from a heart attack, and no matter the verdict, his family would continue to grieve. The cardiologist might "win" if not found at fault, but he might also have a black mark on his record. The hired gun experts couldn't feel entirely great about the work they were doing, though I'm sure they were happy with the money.

The verdict in this case? Not guilty of medical negligence. Even though the patient's outcome was bad, the jury found no fault with the cardiologist's care. Yet he was devastated by the process. He was accustomed to helping people, and now he'd been accused of negligence that had contributed to a man's death. Later, he told me he was thinking of quitting medicine, which would have been yet another loss—in this case, to the field of medicine and all the future patients who might have benefitted from his care. So there really were no winners at all, except maybe the lawyers.

ASSISTANCE IN DYING—PROS AND CONS

Actively assisting a patient in the dying process is an area of continuing discomfort in America. With the advent of palliative care and hospice, most people die comfortably without active medical assistance. Palliative care medicine is a relatively new specialty that does not deal directly with disease but focuses on suffering in a holistic manner. These specialists are called in to help manage patients' symptoms and pain while guiding their overall plan for care. They have strong skills in communication and work with both hospice and non-hospice patients.

Hospice is a special program covered by Medicare and many insurance plans for patients with less than six months to live. The benefits of hospice are many: a 24/7 on-call nurse with home visits; medications, medical equipment, caregiver training and support; spiritual and grief counseling; and volunteers to provide respite for the primary caregiver.

Despite the increasing availability of palliative care and hospice, a growing number of states have passed laws allowing mentally competent but terminal patients to hasten their death by ingesting lethal doses of medication. Do we have a right to die? The case against so-called physician-assisted suicide[1] has been eloquently made by physician, teacher, and author Ira Byock. On the other hand, a book by cardiologist Tom Preston, *Doctor, Please Help Me Die*, presents a strong case for allowing a patient to choose medical assistance in dying.

Let me tell you about an event that pushed these questions straight to the front of my mind.

I entered the exam room as an intravenous catheter was being expertly inserted. The procedure had been explained to me beforehand, and I wanted to be there to comfort my friend in his last moments. Life had been getting difficult for him, the infirmities and pain too severe. The doctor entered the room with an appropriate look of sympathy on his face and reviewed the case, agreeing that my friend's quality of life was severely impaired.

Slowly, sodium pentothal was injected through an IV. I saw a questioning look on my friend's face. He then closed his eyes, slumped on the table, and died. Being unconscious, his breathing stopped almost immediately, then a few minutes later his heartbeat ceased. It all seemed so fast.

I loved my friend, my companion, my dog. We walked in the park or on the beach every morning. He greeted me, my wife, children, and grandchildren each day like long lost buddies. His only goal in life, it seemed, was to protect us.

That day, we grieved. But it didn't feel the same as when I lost my mother and father, or when I'd lost patients. It was a mixture of sadness for our loss, but contentment that his suffering was over and he could have a peaceful end.

Many patients over the years have asked me to ensure a similarly peaceful end. Before hospice and palliative care, patients often felt a terrible loss of control as death approached. Their family members would tell me, "Doctor, my dog was treated more humanely at the end than my father was."

Ironically, my experience with our family dog brought me to ponder how humanely we humans treat one another at the final moments. Do we have lessons to learn?

HELP AT THE END—THE REALITY

At the University Hospital in Madison, Wisc., in 1938, a patient was dying from multiple myeloma, a painful bone cancer that had resulted in several rib and spine fractures. The young interns knew that morphine injections were necessary to control the patient's agony, but they feared they might be blamed for giving a lethal dose. So the interns made a plan. Every hour or so, one of them would give the patient a shot of morphine. This duty was rotated between four or five doctors so that no one would really know who gave the final dose before death. My father told me this story. He had been one of the interns, and he felt strongly that they had taken the right action in a moral sense.

In 1980, I saw a patient I'll call Sam who suffered from a malignancy of the lining of his lungs, related to his work around asbestos in the shipyards during World War II. The asbestos came in bags that the workers dumped into barrels, adding water, then applying the paste to steam pipes in the ship holds for insulation. By the end of a day's work, the men were covered in asbestos dust. Several of Sam's co-workers had already died of the asbestos related cancer—mesothelioma.

In Sam's case, surgery was unsuccessful in that the tumor couldn't be completely removed. Fluid kept building up in Sam's chest, and he was progressively short of breath to the point of gasping. He was unable to lie flat. I could tap off some of the fluid, providing temporary relief, and I tried to scar down the area using a talc solution, but without much success. Sam would come in with his wife, Helen, feeling more discouraged and depressed with each visit. He began asking for frequent refills of his sleeping pills, along with more narcotics. I suspected that he was planning to take a lethal overdose, which was against Washington law at the time—and continues to be against the law in most other states.

"Sam, are you making plans to end your life?"

"I don't know, Doctor, but I want to be able to decide if things get too hard."

I was a member of my hospital's ethics committee, so I decided to present Sam's case to the group. These discussions were only advisory, but always helpful. They are certainly not "death panels." Ethics committees cull the expertise of nurses, doctors, social workers, clergy, consumers, and pharmacists. Ours always engaged in intense discussion. This long before Dr. Kevorkian brought such questions into mainstream conversation, before hospice, and before any state had a Death with Dignity law. After much debate, our committee agreed that while that physician-assisted death was against the law, ethically Sam had the right to self-determination, and to end his life when the suffering was too great.

I saw him several more times. With each visit his condition was worse. Two weeks after our conversation, I got a call that Sam had died at home. The death certificate was delivered to my office the next day. Cause of death assigned by me: mesothelioma—his cancer.

I called Helen a few weeks later with my condolences and asked her if she might be willing to come in and discuss Sam's dying with the ethics committee. "I don't think I can," she replied hesitantly. It was the answer I'd expected.

AGGRESSIVE PALLIATIVE CARE

In the days before hospice, pain management was episodic at best. It's hard to believe that I was never really taught about pain in medical school. Well, that's not entirely true. We were told to make sure patients didn't get "hooked" on narcotics; nurses were drilled similarly. We learned about disease and disease processes, but not much about the full scope of a patient's life in any holistic sense.

Richard was initially referred to me because of masses in his lungs. During the evaluation it became clear that the primary site of his cancer was in the left kidney. A silent cancer, it had spread its tentacles before symptoms ever developed. Now Richard had multiple metastatic tumor growths on his scalp that were excruciatingly painful. Narcotics were necessary. The scalp lesions began to ooze blood and enlarge. Radiation and chemotherapy were ineffective.

I began to receive calls about Richard's narcotic use from the hospice nurse. He was asking for increasing doses of both long-acting and short-acting opiates. The nurses were becoming concerned so we met and discussed the goal in this case: pain relief. Often, a large initial dose of narcotics is used for pain control, leveling off with consistent lower doses to avoid peaks and valleys. The dose we agreed on was "enough to effectively control his pain."

But Richard was now in constant agony and pleading for relief, so his nurses carefully escalated the morphine dosages. That was successful in controlling his pain, and Richard died in three days, much more comfortable but sedated to the point of unconsciousness.

As mentioned above, nowadays a palliative care specialist would consult with hospice on such a case. With multiple specialists involved, the palliative care specialist would help to direct an overall care plan—coordinating treatment and symptom control—while ensuring that the focus remains where it should be: on the patient's needs, whether that means pain management, nausea control or treatment for depression.

Unfortunately, though palliative care centers have been established across the U.S., there simply are not enough palliative care specialists to meet the needs of all patients. Some intensive care specialists also specialize in palliative care medicine[2]—an unusual but promising combination. But until we ramp up the numbers within this growing specialty, palliative care skills should be taught to all medical providers, especially those in primary care.

PULL THE PLUG—NOW!

The voice on the phone was demanding: "Dr. deMaine, you are going to be the attending critical care doctor when our mother is transferred to your hospital today. She needs to be taken off the ventilator and allowed to die. We have been pleading with doctors here at the burn center, but they keep doing more procedures. We want her off life support as soon as she gets there."

I was a bit taken aback since I'd never heard of the patient, let alone that I was destined to be her doctor in the ICU. I told the family to come to the hospital and meet with me when their mother arrived.

Immediately after hanging up, I received the expected call from a transfer coordinator, "We have a patient in the burn unit who is eighty-seven years old. She has 50% third-degree burns and 20% second-degree burns. There have been multiple grafts. The complications have been pneumonia, stroke, heart failure, and acute respiratory distress syndrome. The house staff will fill you in. They think she should stay there, but the family is very unhappy that the patient is suffering through all these treatments."

It's not uncommon for a family to feel left out in critical care decision-making. Sometimes they don't understand that a sick relative may look awful but still have a good chance of recovering. Better communication would help, but it's not a strong suit for many doctors.

I was paged to the ICU when the elderly woman arrived. She had now been on full life support for a month. She'd had multiple burn grafts, and she was unresponsive to verbal or physical stimulus. Her blood pressure was marginal, kidney function poor, liver functions elevated, and chest x-ray diffusely abnormal. If this were a young person, there might have been some hope. But this woman was going progressively downhill. If the patient could talk to us, what would she say?

We all gathered in the conference room—the woman's family, her new RN team, and our hospital social worker. First, we reviewed all the medical facts and a timeline of hospital care to date. Then I outlined the options for further care, including discontinuing it—and the benefits and burdens of each possibility. We discussed the woman's daily life prior to the fire. Her son and daughter, Jerome and Ada, described her as a happy person, yet limited due to arthritis. All her contemporaries had already died, and she had been feeling isolated.

We then discussed her wishes for aggressive life support. She had never signed a living will or designated a Durable Power of Attorney for Health Care. Her husband was deceased, so under Washington state law decision-making authority rested with her two adult children, who needed to agree on the next steps. Both Jerome and Ada were adamant that their mother never would have wanted this kind of aggressive care. She had been ready to "pass on" for some time.

"It's bad enough to die once in a fire," said her son, Jerome. "But dying every day in the ICU is just too much!"

After nearly an hour of discussion, all agreed that the most reasonable course of action was to remove the ventilator. I asked Jerome and Ada to step out of the woman's hospital room. Then I switched off the monitors, made sure she was still unconscious, turned off the ventilator, and removed the endotracheal tube.

Jerome and Ada returned to their mother's bedside and held her hands as she left this world.

The next day, I received a call from the surgical resident in the burn unit, wanting to know about the woman's skin grafts and general status. As gently as possible, I explained that we'd removed life support at the request of the family. The surgical resident was not happy. But it was not his call to make.

DEATH WITH DIGNITY (DWD)

Over the past year, four acquaintances of mine have ingested lethal doses of medication, obtained through a doctor's prescription, in order to control their last moments. Three had cancer, and one had ALS—Lou Gehrig's disease. I was not involved in their medical care, nor as an advisor.

Irene's family was open about her choice. She was ninety, frail, and very tired. The diagnosis was an acute form of leukemia. "I'm not interested in chemotherapy," said Irene. "Just let me go quickly."

After she was gone, Irene's family held an open meeting at the care facility to discuss Irene's choice to die. Ninety friends and acquaintances attended. The family spoke of her wish for medical aid in dying and wanted others to know that she'd had a peaceful end to her life.

Eighty-eight-year-old Gordon called me to say goodbye the night before he ended his life. He had advanced pancreatic cancer and had been living with a drainage tube placed in his destroyed gallbladder. He couldn't get comfortable, even with help from hospice. Sleeping was all but impossible. A scientist by training, Gordon wanted control at the end. His doctor helped him obtain the medication, and a nurse friend helped him mix it. With his family present, Gordon sat in his living room chair, drank the medication, and within five minutes was gone.

Matt was a retired pathologist. He didn't realize that he had advanced prostate cancer until it spread to his spine, causing paralysis. He was told he likely had less than six months to live, and he didn't like the idea of spending that much time in a nursing home. Matt was alert and rational. He wanted to be in control of his life (and death). I was called to witness his signature on the necessary forms, and the nursing home did not object because what Matt did was lawful in Washington. He died peacefully.

Nancy had advanced ALS. She'd suffered progressive weakness and difficulty with speech and swallowing. She'd also had several pneumonias and felt each time that she was suffocating. Nancy's family was very private so the details of her death were not widely known. But it's likely that it occurred at her vacation home. Her husband simply told me, "Now she's at peace."

I offer these four real-life examples to present the kinds of scenarios in which Death with Dignity laws are used. Oregon led the way with legislation in 1997 allowing physicians to prescribe lethal medication in certain cases. Washington's Death with Dignity Act followed in 2009, passing with 59% of the vote. Eight states and Washington, D.C., currently have death with dignity statutes. California's end of life option act went into effect in 2016. All of these laws are similar: if a person is confirmed to have less than six months to live, their physician may order oral medications to end their lives. There must be a written request by the person, a waiting period, and a mental health assessment. Most importantly, the patient must administer the lethal medication to himself; no one may assist.

Initially, I had some concerns about the potential abuse of these so-called Death with Dignity laws. As more of us reach advanced age and the pressure to conserve health resources mounts, we need to ensure that individuals are making autonomous, well-informed choices. We also need to ensure that affordable health care, plus superb hospice and palliative care, are available to these very ill people.

Currently, only 1 in 500 deaths in Washington occur via the Death with Dignity route.

In my practice, I cared for many patients at the end, few of whom ever invoked the DWD option. Instead, I saw more terminal patients referred to hospice, fewer hospital deaths, and more comfort for the patient and their loved ones. Often, that is their greatest wish. So, despite my worries, Death with Dignity laws ironically seem to have made the medical and nursing profession step up to provide more sensitive end-of-life care.

Is that name too euphemistic? Does it imply that other kinds of deaths are undignified? Those who oppose the DWD acts call them physician-assisted suicide. And the Catholic Church[3] has been particularly resistant, perceiving these laws as evidence of a "culture of death" in our society. Some Catholics believe that suffering is redemptive, and that we should not interfere with the life force in any way, a position that must be acknowledged.

These are sensitive issues, and disagreement around them will not disappear any time soon. Either way, "death with dignity" might be more accurately described as patient choice in dying—certainly, that would be more realistic.

Medical Assistance in Dying (MAID) is what they call it in Canada, which has liberalized its laws around end-of-life decisions. In Canada, MAID laws now allow physicians to directly administer lethal drugs either orally or intravenously to hasten death in certain patients with "grievous and irremediable conditions."[4] The other crucial difference, compared to our laws, is that there is no requirement for the person to have a terminal prognosis of six months or less.

Should there be limits on our autonomy to choose? Where do we draw that line? Controversy around this question has even spilled over into the use of advance directives, with some suggesting that such planning is tantamount to a "death panel."[5] It is my hope, however, that the ethics around an individual's right to choose what is done to his or her own body continues to inform our laws.

DEATH BY VOLUNTARY CESSATION OF FLUIDS AND NUTRITION

My friend Carol called me about her husband. Perhaps she was seeking reassurance that they were doing the right thing, now that Carol's role was helping her husband to die. John had descended into dementia, but he was still in the early stages—enough to recognize what was happening. "I'm becoming some kind of sub-human," he said, commenting on the progressive loss of his mind. "I'm no longer myself."

John often forgot appointments. He had trouble with sequential tasks, and was becoming withdrawn. He had progressed rapidly from mild cognitive impairment to early dementia, and his prognosis was poor. He knew he might live another two to four years in this state, and was frightened. A scientist trained in physics, John had always loved problem-solving. He had five patents in his name. The university where he'd earned his PhD repeatedly recognized him for outstanding teaching.

"I don't want to become someone I'm not," John told Carol. "I don't see any point living with this. I just don't want to go there."

Carol was shocked. She was loath to lose him, but she knew she would support his decision. They'd had deep conversations about his fear of losing mental capacity, and they'd contacted medical providers about physician-assisted dying.

But John did not qualify for this because he did not have a terminal prognosis of six months or less. There are networks of people who attempt to skirt Death with Dignity laws by engineering the end-of-life by other means. John found them creepy.

"I don't like the idea of my head in a bag hooked up to a tank of helium or nitrogen," he said. "There's got to be a legal option."

A friend introduced them to the concept of VSED, which stands for Voluntary Stopping Eating and Drinking. They did some research and, with some difficulty, found a doctor who would guide them through this choice. Carol hated the whole process. But she kept coming back to the reality of John's disease and his right to choose his own end.

VSED deserves more understanding and discussion. Law Professor Thaddeus Mason Pope notes that it is well established law that we can refuse medical treatment including fluids and nutrition. He lays it all out in his excellent article, "Voluntarily Stopping Eating and Drinking Is Legal—and Ethical—for Terminally Ill Patients Looking to Hasten Death."[6]

After much discussion, the day arrived when VSED began for John. The first problem was extreme dry mouth, then thirst—then uncomfortable thirst. Carol swabbed John's mouth, as she'd been directed, and John took no sips of water. He was on low-dose sedatives to suppress the discomfort, and his doctor visited John at home to check that all was proceeding as planned. John read, watched *I Love Lucy* videos, and talked about his life. The couple had no immediate family, but close friends called and visited. By the fourth day, John began to have periods of deep sleep with deep breathing. His body was dry and not difficult to care for. Finally, on the ninth day, as Carol put it, John gave up his earthly body and claimed his beautiful spiritual one in the next life.

My own father went through a more common version of the same. At age ninety-three, he gradually, naturally, began to eat less. Cognitively, he was slowing, and eventually, he began refusing to eat anything at all. This was followed by minimal fluid intake, though he would accept sips of water. To me, his was an example of what I'd call natural VSED—the body simply wearing out as a result of old age. There would have been no benefit to IV fluids or tube feeding. My dad had a right to die without "medicalizing" his death, and he slipped away peacefully.

Utilizing VSED allows many more individuals than are covered by physician aid-in-dying laws to end life on their terms. The process is gradually garnering wider discussion. Both Diane Rehm's book *On My Own* and Phyllis Schacter's *Choosing to Die: A Personal Story: Elective Death by Voluntarily Stopping Eating and Drinking (VSED) in the Face of Degenerative Disease* poignantly reveal what it is to become an advocate and caregiver to a spouse descending into dementia. The first international VSED conference was held at the Seattle University School of Law in 2016, with an emphasis on ethical, legal, family, clinical and religious concerns.

IS SUICIDE EVER RATIONAL?

Beyond the protocols for MAID and VSED, some argue that suicide may, at times, be rational. This is a difficult subject for me. Two of my friends killed themselves with handguns in recent years. One had a failing business venture. The other likely had a poorly managed manic-depressive disorder. In retrospect, it is clear that both of my friends had shown warning signs of depression. (The main risk factors for senior suicides are depression, debility, access to deadly means, and disconnectedness, known as "the four Ds."). The scars left behind after deaths like these remain deeply imbedded in the psyches of surviving families and communities—a painful legacy.

Suicidal gestures are highest for young adults undergoing a crisis. But suicide rates are increasing across all age groups, particularly among the elderly, who commit suicide with a frequency more than four times the age-adjusted national average.[7] Suicide is now the tenth leading cause of death[8] in the United States, more than double the number of homicides.

Suicide which is always tragic and often preventable. But can it ever be rational? Kaiser News reports that small groups of seniors meet openly to discuss this question.[9] A few hundred seniors each year commit suicide when transitioning either to or from long-term care facilities. It's unclear how many were clear-headed when they made this choice. But it appears they wanted to be able to end their lives when circumstances came to feel unbearable. Among the elderly a major concern is the fear of progressive dementia, or an illness, that will seriously limit their ability to enjoy living—even if their disease is not terminal. "Heck, I've lived a full life. I'm basically falling apart," they say. "There's nothing to look forward to so I'm ready to die."

This concept of "rational suicide" is worrisome to me. Dr. Yeates Conwell,[10] a psychiatrist at the University of Rochester and leading expert on elder suicide, feels that widespread ageism is particularly dangerous in this regard. If ageism begins to normalize suicide among the elderly, it will profoundly change the way we look at aging and dying.

But then there are depictions of this struggle through films like *Amour*. If you haven't seen it, I hope you get the chance. *Amour* starts and ends with love, but not in the usual, youthful fashion of a Hollywood romance. It focuses on death after a life of love, longtime care, and, finally, suffering.

The story begins in the apartment of two aging musicians. As the wife suffers a series of strokes, her mind and her will to live erode. Her life becomes agonizing, and her caregiver husband is exhausted. This painful circumstance, common to many real-life couples handling illness on their own, was dramatized so beautifully that *Amour* won the 2013 Academy Award for Best Foreign Language Film.

Was it reasonable for the wife to attempt suicide? Was it OK for her to make her husband promise never to take her back to the hospital? Could the couple's daughter have been more supportive? What happens as the loving caregiver is finally at wits end? *Amour* left me full of lingering questions about the choices this couple made, yet admiration for the love between them as they navigated the process of dying.

In real life, sadly, the death of an elderly couple can be violent and abrupt. Not long ago, in a nursing home near me, two residents in their nineties were found dead in their apartment, both from gunshot wounds, in an apparent murder-suicide. About twenty older Americans die in this manner each week in the United States, according to estimates.[11] I see nothing loving in those situations. Typically, a controlling husband shoots his wife in her sleep, then turns the gun on himself. There is often a history of domestic abuse. Most commonly, the underlying issue is depression. Families, physicians, and caregivers need to be on alert and unafraid to ask about mood changes and suicidal thoughts. There is no easy solution, but we can all reach out and, if there are concerns about potential self-harm, call 1-800-273-TALK (8255).

There certainly are actions that physicians and loved ones can take to help before things get that dire. We need to address loneliness, depression, spousal abuse, cognitive changes, and housing stability for the aging. We need to better ensure access to caregivers and loved ones. In my own retirement community, a friend observed, "I'm sure we live longer and happier lives here because of our connected community of people." I believe this is true.

To my mind, the concept of rational suicide remains nuanced; it is certainly not black or white. For those who are not terminally ill, choosing VSED could be seen as an example of rational suicide, as it is a conscientious decision made not out of depression or other mental illness, but as an option against enduring a deteriorated quality of life. For the terminally ill with severe suffering, I consider MAID a rational response, as long as patients are screened for mental health and legal safeguards are in place.

But MAID and VSED remain uncommon. With the advent of hospice and palliative care, most of us will die naturally, hopefully without great discomfort, and ideally in a manner that allows for healing and a positive legacy for those we leave behind.

DOCTOR, I WANT TO DIE

On call one day, I was urgently summoned to the E.R. to tend to a young man I'll call Dan, who was suddenly paralyzed. He was the only one in the family who had eaten his wife's home-canned spin-ach, and he'd contracted acute botulism poisoning. After rapid intu-bation, Dan was transferred to the ICU for ongoing ventilator and supportive care. We gave him an anti-toxin as soon as we could get it.

Sue, his wife, was devastated. She knew she was responsible for the terrible mistake. She was so relieved that their two children didn't like spinach!

The anti-toxin had no measurable benefit. Dan required tube feeding, an air bed to prevent skin ulcers, close monitoring of his ventilator, and vigilance against infections. He was awake but couldn't move or breathe without support. Sue remained with him constantly, and their kids, ages two and four, were allowed to visit.

It was going to take a few months for Dan's paralysis to clear. But his prognosis was good if we could avoid complications, par-ticularly infection. After four weeks, he began to be able to com-municate. When he did, Dan made it clear that his dependence on a ventilator and ongoing need for full body care made life no lon-ger worth living—even if he might someday recover. He wanted to be allowed to die. "Take me off this machine and let me go," Dan said.

I asked a psychiatrist to see him, and Dan was judged mentally competent, not clinically depressed. The psychiatrist did note, however, that Dan did not seem to realize he was going to get better. He simply could not see beyond the jail of his bed and ventilator. After discussing the case with my colleagues, I told Dan that because of his excellent prognosis we couldn't agree to remove the ventilator. Generally, on ethical matters patient autonomy car-ries the day. But in this case, our Ethics Committee agreed with a stance that, technically, violated that rule because other ethical principles—beneficence and non-malfeasance (do no harm)—were the ones that seemed most appropriate. We continued with the ventilator, despite Dan's wishes.

He demanded to see a lawyer. But the lawyer went along with what Dan's wife and medical team were saying; there was no way to get a court order or guardianship under these circumstances, he explained. There was some precedent for what Dan asked, I should note. In a famous "wrongful life" case, the U.S. Airforce pilot Dax Cowart[12] begged to be allowed to die after being severely burned in a propane gas explosion and losing his hands and sight. His wishes were not honored. Subsequently, Cowart became an attorney promoting patients' rights to refuse treatment. Nonetheless, our ethics committee felt we needed to advocate for Dan's healthy future. In fact, there were legal risks on either course—withdraw life support from a basically healthy person, or save his life by treating him without his consent.

Dan survived, returning to his life as a husband, father, and productive citizen. Yet when I saw him in my office months later, I found him still conflicted.

"So how do you feel about our keeping you going against your wishes?" I asked.

He paused. "Well, Doc," Dan said, "I'm happy to be alive, but there's a part of me that's still pissed off."

Was Dan's temporary suffering worth his ultimate survival? The answer to that depends on whom you ask. And he's hardly the only person struggling with this kind of conflict. Years ago, a lawyer friend of mine endured an extensive chest wall resection for lung cancer. He suffered terribly during radiation and chemotherapy, but five years later was alive and pain free—a rare cure. Yet my friend told me he'd wanted to die during his months of agony—in fact, he wished he had died. The suffering remains seared on his memory, and with that ghost looming, he felt that survival was not worth it.

DO EVERYTHING?

The room was darkened, the parents distraught, and the social worker sat quietly as I opened the door to Room 202 on the medical ward. My pager had buzzed me early that Sunday morning, as I was on call for pulmonary consults. A fourteen-year-old boy,

Noah, was dying. His history was that of a previously healthy youngster who had a widespread metastatic osteosarcoma of the femur. Bone cancer. But it had spread. An x-ray showed multiple masses throughout both of Noah's lungs. He was struggling to breathe, even with an oxygen mask.

The surprising part of the story is that Noah had never been treated. There were procedures, including chemotherapy and amputation, that might have made a difference. But Noah's parents believed he could be healed by prayer.

Early on, Noah's medical team had tried to get a court order for treatment, or at least the appointment of a legal guardian who could advocate for medical intervention. But those efforts had come too late to prevent Noah's now rapid downhill course. I must admit that I wasn't happy about this consult because it seemed like there was nothing I could do. I was an impotent adjunct to a sad and frustrating story.

When I walked into Noah's room, I found him looking emaciated and pale. With a weak smile, he said his main concern was trouble breathing. His lung exam showed abnormal crackling sounds, and his heart rate was fast at 130 with a thready pulse.

As I began to discuss options for addressing his breathing problems, I discovered that no one had discussed the "code status" with Noah or his family. In other words, if the boy's breathing or heart beat ceased, would we do CPR? That route made no sense to me, considering Noah's prognosis, nor did a ventilator in the ICU. The question was how to broach this with his family.

We all met—the parents, a social worker, nurse, respiratory therapist, and me—in a conference area near Noah's room. I reviewed the medical facts and let his mother and father know that I thought their son's remaining time was very limited, perhaps only hours or days. They didn't seem surprised. They'd watched Noah go downhill, while still hoping and praying for a miracle. Yet when the prospect of using a ventilator was raised, they said they wanted everything possible to be done. This position perplexed me, since they'd previously been so invested in prayer as

Noah's primary treatment. But here we were: with a terminal case, a teenager, and two very sad parents.

When families say they want "everything" done, it's usually time for a discussion to explore precisely what they mean by that word. I was candid with Noah's parents. I needed to make sure they understood that a ventilator would require an uncomfortable tube in Noah's throat and heavy sedation. It would certainly increase their son's suffering. I explained this as gently as I could and let them know that we would not do CPR if his heart stopped. I felt neither a ventilator nor CPR would have any benefit.

This is what we now call seeking "informed assent."[13] Instead of requesting a family's consent to initiate invasive life support, the physician explains that he is *not* offering resuscitative intervention. It's not a set-in-stone ruling. If a family disagrees, we talk about it. But most often, by the time a case gets to this point, people understand, and informed assent spares them the burden of making a DNR decision. It is very rare for a doctor to unilaterally sign a DNR order.

Yet we did not want Noah or his family to feel abandoned.

"Doctor," said the respiratory therapist, "how about the Bird Respirator to support his breathing?"

This turned out to be a wonderful compromise. The Bird Respirator, a device that can support breathing and deliver oxygen, was invented by Dr. Forrest Bird during the polio epidemics. Today, we'd call it non-invasive ventilation. It is relatively low tech and similar in concept to a CPAP machine. By using the Bird Respirator, we could help Noah breathe without needing to transfer him to the ICU. Essentially, we were using it to offer palliative care without labeling it that way. Some might argue that I was being overly paternalistic, but I felt compelled to advocate for a peaceful death for this boy.

Several hours later, with his respirator attached, Noah passed away comfortably. His parents felt that everything had been done and were grateful that no one chastised them for their belief in faith healing.

ETHICS ON THIN ICE

As in the case above, doctors sometimes walk a delicate line in honoring our vow to do no harm while operating in a manner that is medically sound. Consider the case of Shirley. Every two weeks she was taken by ambulance from her nursing home to our E.R. for blood transfusions. These transfusions were keeping her alive. The problem was that every time Shirley was moved she decompensated. Her Alzheimer's was severe. She no longer recognized her family. At eighty-three, she was slowly dying.

Shirley had aplastic anemia. Her bone marrow could no longer make enough red blood cells to keep her alive. Medications to stimulate red blood cell production were no longer working and, by medical protocol, Shirley's transfusions could not be given in a nursing home so she arrived every two weeks to get two units of packed red blood cells. Poor Shirley often screamed when stuck with the needles. Then she'd require sedative medications and wind up getting admitted. It was kind of a medical merry-go-round, though not so merry.

This time, I was on call. Shirley had had perhaps ten admissions already. I didn't feel the transfusions were extending her life in any beneficial way. They appeared to be making her miserable and prolonging her death so I gathered her husband and children for a discussion about end-of-life plans.

We set aside an hour late one afternoon. The social worker who had been working with Shirley's family joined us, as did her primary nurse. We reviewed Shirley's medical history and asked the family to fill in a few missing details, encouraging their participation. There were many moments of sadness and some expressions of "if only." But, in general, the family seemed to have a realistic understanding of Shirley's poor outlook and even worse quality of life.

Then we discussed various scenarios around the issue of more blood transfusions. When I brought up the option of hospice—and no further transfusions—Shirley's husband, Morrie, jumped out of his chair, very agitated. "This is like Dachau!" he shouted. The room was silent as he stomped out.

The others kept talking. They noted that Morrie had early Alzheimer's himself and required ever-increasing supervision. Yet they wanted to honor his feelings. Shirley had never completed an advance directive, but her family felt certain that she wouldn't have wanted to continue living in her current state. Given this impasse, I suggested a one-on-one meeting between Morrie and myself.

The next day, we sat down to talk. Morrie was no longer upset. In fact, he seemed eager to discuss Shirley's care. In broaching the ethics of the situation, I explained that Shirley's blood transfusions might actually be harming her.

"You know, I agree with you," he said, to my great surprise.

"Why is that?" I asked.

"She might get AIDS!"

With Morrie fixated on his fear of AIDS, the family determined that there would be no further transfusions (even though AIDS-contaminated blood was not an issue). Hospice was begun and provided wonderful support to Morrie and the family as Shirley went downhill and died peacefully in her nursing home several weeks later.

Perhaps it seems cavalier, ethically speaking, to have stumbled upon this way of getting Morrie to agree with me and the rest of the family. But his decision-making appeared impaired, and the "do no harm" principle was my primary guide. Still, this case was anything but textbook. As I've said, medicine is an art as well as a science and, very often, a delicate balancing act between the two.

PLEASE, PLEASE LET ME DIE

Many times, Erik's wife had warned him: "Stay off ladders, dear. Leave it to someone younger." But Erik was a spry seventy-two, and he had been cleaning his gutters for many years. He had a sturdy, twenty-five-foot extension ladder and decades of experience as an athlete. He wasn't about to slow down without a good reason.

On an unusually crisp November day, Erik laid his ladder against the house. It shouldn't be hard to clear the soggy maple and oak leaves, he thought, securing the footing and donning rubber gloves.

How long was Erik up there, tossing matted leaves toward the recycling bin two stories below in his yard? Impossible to say. Later, all he could recall was an ache that started slowly in his neck and left arm, then ballooned into a crushing chest pain that took his breath away and threw him backwards onto the ground.

Erik awoke in the Medic One ambulance, trying to pull the tube from his throat. But he was immobilized. He thought of Kafka's *Metamorphosis*. Was he Gregor Samsa, awakening as a giant insect trapped on his back, struggling with his new existence? Was this real?

Erik's wife, Gerta, had found him unconscious at the foot of the ladder, barely breathing. The medics arrived within two minutes, found Erik to be in ventricular fibrillation and applied CPR, then shocked his heart back into normal rhythm. Erik's color "pinked up" as his circulation returned, and the medics rushed him to the trauma center.

When Erik woke, he felt no pain. In fact, he felt nothing at all. He tried to move his arms and legs but couldn't. He saw Gerta crying at his bedside. This a former athlete lay there, a helpless lump. He couldn't believe it.

An MRI scan showed that Erik had severed his cervical spine at the C1 level. He was now quadriplegic and would need to stay on a breathing machine indefinitely. Happily, he had no brain damage because CPR had been successfully started within a few minutes of his fall. But Erik was devastated.

It was the fall, he knew. Gerta had been right. Why didn't he listen?

The couple had been successful entrepreneurs in high tech, and they knew how to get things done. They also had resources for the very best care. Erik began an intensive program to get mobile as soon as possible. He underwent a tracheotomy, and Gerta bought a specially equipped wheel chair with a battery powered ventilator. A custom breathing tube allowed Erik to talk in a stuttering manner, a major step toward self-sufficiency, and the electric wheelchair could be controlled by Erik's exhalations so he became mobile. Gerta had the house remodeled, allowing her husband to navigate throughout the main floor, out the door, onto a ramp, and all the way down to the swimming pool (now barricaded). Gerta was expending a huge amount of energy trying to make Erik as happy as possible.

Dutifully, he went through rehabilitation, but became progressively more discouraged. Erik hated the daily massages to prevent sores, tone his muscles, and get his bowels moving. He required periodic enemas and a catheter into his bladder. None of it was as miserable as the bouts of recurrent pneumonia. Each time, Erik would struggle to breathe and require suctioning from his trachea because he couldn't cough effectively. The first year, there were five trips to the E.R., two requiring a hospital stay.

In the second year, Erik's pneumonias worsened, and I knew he was struggling emotionally too. Gerta was sitting with us when Erik clearly said, "I don't think it's worth it."

"Erik, you can't mean that!" she said, plainly shocked. "There's so much more that can be done, and I can't think of living without you."

He backed off. But when we spoke later, alone, Erik returned to the topic. "Look doctor, enough is enough. This isn't living. Do I have to go on this way?"

"Erik, are you down? Are you depressed?"

"Wouldn't you be?" he said, with more than a touch of scorn.

I asked my favorite practical psychiatrist for an assessment. He found that Erik was thinking clearly and not clinically depressed. He wasn't suicidal per se, but saw no future in continuing on.

I asked Erik to tell me why he felt this way.

"First, I'm no longer functioning as a man," he said. "I'm worsening, have no chance of recovering, and am a burden to my wife. I'm serious—I should have the right to decide."

Gerta, distraught, pushed Erik to go on. So he did. But in the third year following his accident, Erik had yet another bout of severe pneumonia and landed in the ICU. At the bedside, I heard him make himself absolutely clear: "I'm ready to meet my maker and finally be at peace."

Still, Gerta resisted. "I just don't want to lose him," she kept saying. "He means everything to me."

A social worker spent hours talking with her, and slowly Gerta came to believe that it was kinder to support her husband's wish to die than force him to go on. Legally, it can be termed "assault" when medical procedures are forced on a person. We have the right to refuse treatment even if we might die without it. Gerta reluctantly came to understand that Erik did indeed have the right to refuse further ventilator support.

After further conferencing with Gerta, the social worker, and the ICU nurses, we sedated Erik with small doses of morphine and removed his ventilator. He died peacefully with Gerta at his bedside.

Erik's choice was one that I will long remember. Did I do the right thing? Didn't people like Steven Hawking live for years on ventilators? Didn't Christopher Reeves (Superman) struggle even more than Erik before succumbing to a similar injury? Being a doctor can confer god-like powers on a person. What's best? Is there a clear right or wrong? I felt my obligation was to support my patient's wishes, even if that meant discontinuing artificial means of life support. There's a well-known quote in medicine from Dr. Francis Peabody:[14] "One of the essential qualities of the clinician is interest in humanity, for the secret of the care of the patient is in caring for the patient."

FLAWED ETHICS—THE DIE AT 75 PLAN

In 2014, Ezekiel Emanuel wrote an article for the *Atlantic* provocatively titled *"Why I Hope to Die at 75."*[45] His argument posited that society and families—all of us—are better off when nature takes its course swiftly. As an oncologist and ethicist, he says he speaks for himself. But the clear implication is that it's best for everyone if we avoid the consequences of aging and declining health. Emanuel says he will eschew all medical tests or therapeutics after age seventy-five. By that point, he argues, the productive years of life are over and accomplishments should be complete. Prolonging the discomfort of aging is pointless, he says, and something he'd like to avoid.

Emanuel wrote that his family disagrees with his wishes. I hope he can find someone to follow them and respect his autonomy. But I'm with the family. What if he comes in with an hangnail that gets infected and could, technically, threaten his life? At seventy-four, he'd take an antibiotic, but decline it the following year?

When I recently gave my talk "Your Life, Your Choices" at a couple of senior communities, we discussed Emanuel's piece. The average age among my audience was nearly eighty. Most of these residents were still semi-independent. Many had lost spouses and had some degree of declining health. A depressing scenario in Emanuel's view—unacceptable, actually. Yet these folks were active—in their faith groups, with their grandchildren, swimming, singing, line dancing, playing tennis or golf, performing in bands or quartets, and enjoying each other's company. None of them felt they should have died five years earlier! They had thought through end-of-life options, and many had POLST forms saying they would never want CPR but would accept removal of an appendix or replacement of an old hip.

I think Emanuel's response to aging is exaggerated, maybe extreme. But I agree that we need to think carefully about prolonging the dying process as we near the end. It's a question of ethics, in my view. There are delights in being old while still functional. True, we are unlikely to win a Nobel Prize at that age. But does this mean we should give up the joy of attending a grandchild's concert? Or going up to the lake cabin once more with the family? Or traveling to Alaska, singing old favorites, volunteering at a food bank, or going to the opera? There is no age cutoff for enjoying family, friends, and the pleasures of life. Emanuel says he does not support "death with dignity" laws, but by declining to take an antibiotic after age seventy-five, wouldn't the result be the same?

Using a cane, walker, or wheelchair does not preclude having an enjoyable life. There can be spiritual growth and even newfound love as we experience loss. Personally, I believe that rekindling an old friendship at seventy or eighty or ninety is more important than climbing Mt. Kilimanjaro.

So, Dr. Emanuel, as I write this at age eighty-one, I think your ethics around aging are at best cloudy, based on fear of loss and touched with ageism. Yes, there are questions around intelligent use of medical resources, exorbitant public costs, and "getting out of the way" for the next generation. But with my new corneas, I can drive safely again and play tennis doubles with my eighty-five-year-old friends twice a week. Should I have resigned myself to going blind at seventy-five?

You are a healthy fifty-eight today, and I likely won't be around by the time you reach seventy-four. But I'd love to see a rewrite of your article around that time.

REFLECTIONS

I *learned to expect the unexpected in my medical practice. Dull moments were few. In these eclectic reflections I touch on the COVID-19 pandemic, common and uncommon diseases, the discovery of a previously unknown syndrome, health care costs, and strange things that happen in hospitals that you never hear about.*

SPIRITUALITY AND THE DOCTOR

William would come to see me every three months for his COPD (Chronic Obstructive Pulmonary Disease). We would chat about his illness, his meds, and his grief. He had lost his wife a few years back, and after fifty-two years of marriage he found it very hard to be without her.

On one visit he said, "Doctor deMaine, can I tell you something—and promise you won't think I'm crazy?"

"Sure."

"Well, my wife and I always had a favorite restaurant where we'd go for our dinner on Sundays. Let me tell you why I still go there. I wear my old tie and coat and sit in our favorite booth. And I swear that I see her. Her image is perfect, younger and smiling. She looks beautiful. She doesn't really communicate except with the smile—which seems to me to say that she's waiting for me."

Other patients related different views. A very sweet British lady told me on an office visit that she had been a widow now for six months.

"That's sad," I said. "Do you believe in an afterlife?"

"Of course," she replied.

"How about marriage in heaven?"

"Yes."

Trying to tie this together I said, "That's wonderful. Perhaps you and your husband can spend eternity together."

She paused, tilted her head, and said, "Well, I might play the field a bit first!"

Views of an afterlife vary from none to quite fanciful. Harvard theologian Huston Smith in the Ingersoll Lecture "Intimations of Immortality"[1] highlights those of the Swedish scientist and theologian Emmanuel Swedenborg, who had great influence on the New England transcendentalists and many others. Theologians seem to struggle with what "heaven" might be, but less academic folks often see it as a spiritual extension of this life, where they will joyfully reunite with loved ones.

Helen Keller with her blindness and deafness was, in those senses, cut off from the world. Yet she was a great student of the Bible and became very influenced by Swedenborg's writings. She wrote: "By 'church' [Swedenborg] did not mean an ecclesiastical organization, but a spiritual fellowship of thoughtful men and women who spend their lives for a service to mankind that outlasts them. He called it a civilization that was to be born of a healthy, universal religion—goodwill, mutual understanding, service from each to all, regardless of dogma or ritual."[2]

Mark Twain's views were more irreverent: "Go to Heaven for the climate; go to Hell for the company."[3] In *Captain Stormfield's Visit to Heaven*,[4] he further described his views of life after death: "...Now you just remember this—heaven is as blissful and lovely as it can be; but it's just the busiest place you ever heard of. There ain't any idle people here after the first day. Singing hymns and waving palm branches through all eternity is pretty when you hear about it in the pulpit, but it's as poor a way to put in valuable time as a body could contrive. It would just make a heaven of warbling ignoramuses, don't you see?"

The formerly agnostic neurosurgeon Eben Alexander III published a rather astounding book, *Proof of Heaven*, in which he describes his experience of the spiritual world while in a coma and near death. This is difficult for me to explain away, though some of his readers will remain unconvinced. Perhaps true "proof" might hamper our free will to choose what to believe —which would make us less human.

My education along these lines came through my days as a student at Bryn Athyn College. For two years, I was immersed in the teachings of Plato, Aristotle, and others thinkers, including Swedenborg. My studies held that we possess two capabilities that make us uniquely human: freedom and rationality. At Bryn Athyn, we were told to apply these lessons to life. It was heady stuff for a twenty-year-old, but increasingly meaningful as I aged. I hope more young physicians are exposed to a liberal arts education—medicine, after all, is much more than science.

Do these thoughts about an afterlife carry over into medical practice? Since we are all in some sense spiritual beings, it seems logical for physicians to deal with the whole person, particularly around a time of crisis or death. I am not one who thinks a chosen few believers have some sort of "inside track" or die easier than atheists. I've had confirmed non-believers in my care who comfortably passed away believing "that was that." They appeared to be good people who had led good lives.

But others want to talk, are afraid, or have regrets. Nowadays, all hospitals and most nursing homes get regular visits from ministers, rabbis, imams, and priests. Doctors of course, must respect all beliefs and understand boundaries. One pulmonologist I knew of would ask patients to pray with him before he did their procedures—clearly a boundary violation. (His group rightly let him go.) And although I loved having philosophical discussions with patients, I always tried to approach these talks from their interests and comfort levels.

On the other hand, I once heard from a patient in Loveland, Colo., who had this to say: "Some years ago I was evaluated by a neurologist because of frequent headaches and other symptoms.

He had me get an MRI and did a battery of other tests. Good news! Nothing scary on my scan and everything else appeared normal. But he knew I was having problems for some reason. I'll never forget that as the appointment came to an end, he gently asked if I would consider praying with him. We bowed our heads and he led us in a humble prayer asking for God's help in healing me. I had never had a doctor do this. I was so touched that, to this doctor, I was more than just an appointment on his schedule. I appreciated this gesture. Maybe some patients would be put off, but he certainly didn't push it at me, and it felt like a full service stop."

Spiritual beliefs can be, and in my opinion should be, an important part of the conversation when we communicate our choices about care, particularly when we are facing the end of our lives. I encouraged my students, interns, and residents to become comfortable with this and not avoid these areas. Healing and caring occur on many levels.

THE COVID-19 PANDEMIC

For decades, heart disease and cancer accounted for the majority of deaths in high income countries. But in early 2020, the world was suddenly turned upside down. No one, of any age, was immune to a new strain of coronavirus that touched off worldwide panic, at a scale unknown since the influenza epidemic of 1918.[5] COVID-19 infections were spreading due to the enemy we could not see. The SARS-CoV-2 microscopic virus captured our psyches as well as our bodies. It spawned not just one sprawling story, but millions of individual stories of loss, fear, and grief in a new dystopian state.

It was the mom who worked at the grocery store and feared for the health of herself and her children. The child who had lost his teacher, friend, or parent. It was the E.R. doctor who'd never thought of her work as a war zone, never known such fear for her staff or her own safety, as she moved to the bedside of yet another sick patient, without a fresh mask or gown. It was the hair salon owner—how would she survive the resulting economic shutdown, even with government support? It was the medic racing from one crisis to another; the daughter whose mother was one of many found dead at a nursing home; the patient surrounded by strangers in that foreign country known as the ICU. It was loved ones unable to be at the bedside. Nurses weeping with shock at the loss of a vibrant young colleague. It was New York City honoring its health workers by applauding them nightly from apartment windows. Lines of people descending on food banks. Essential workers sleeping in their cars.

On a Zoom call with critical care physicians across Washington, I could feel their worry as cases poured into hospitals from nearby nursing homes. There were a million questions to be answered. But beyond those of COVID-19's transmission and treatment, I kept thinking about another looming concern: the quality of these patients' last moments of life.

Ventilators were scarce suddenly, so who should get one? (And who should not?) COVID-19 brought medical ethics to the forefront of everyday conversations in a way I'd never seen before. Years before at a medical conference, I'd participated in a simulated conversation around similar quandaries. In that hypothetical, there were fifteen of us who needed a new life saving drug, but only ten treatments available. Would we divide the medication equally so that everyone got at least some? Should we draw straws? Designate the "more critical" patients for priority? Or give the treatment to those who could pay the most? Should we consider the age, health, social contribution, or societal worth of each patient?

COVID-19 made these exercises starkly real. Suddenly people were having end-of-life conversations hurriedly, in hospital hallways. Some families elected to ensure that their sick relations were simply as comfortable as possible until the end, forgoing potential treatments. Wherever families landed in these discussions, the reality of dying—whenever it might be—became present to a wide swath of Americans in ways it had not been before.

Each of us has been pressed to find ways of increasing our resilience. Each of us has been forced to adapt. Some have found that talking regularly with loved ones is more important to their lives than they'd realized. Others have thrown themselves into exercise, meditation, or work. Some have become newly philosophical about adversity. Others have found relief through activities like volunteerism. Writers write. Gardeners garden.

Whatever our response, the pandemic has made the prospect of death a much more urgent reality and one that has forced more of us to think about its practicalities. It has naturally forced a confrontation with the meaning of loss. But in so doing, it has also brought many of us closer together.

CE N'EST PAS SI DIFFICILE
(IT'S NOT SO DIFFICULT)

The coronavirus pandemic, among its many lessons, underscored the ease with which infectious diseases can spread. You might think that at this point in medical history, we would have learned this well. But the realities of MRSA and other so-called superbugs show that all of us—including doctors—still have a long way to go on procedures to control the spread of infection.

A young doctor looked spiffy in his white doctor's jacket and tie. He saw and touched twelve patients on rounds that morning. He washed his hands only occasionally, did not don gloves, did not wipe his stethoscope with antiseptic, and had not changed his white coat for two days. He would be horrified to know that MRSA (virulent staph bacteria), C diff, and E Coli could be found on his white coat, fingers, and even his stethoscope.

A word here about C Diff, which is becoming increasingly prevalent in U.S. hospitals. Doctors understood that antibiotics were killing off the normal bowel bacteria we need, and that this sometimes resulted in serious illness or death. But the exact cause wasn't pinpointed until 1978.[6]

Bacteria called Clostridium Difficile (C Diff) proved to be the culprit. It's hard to grow in a lab but produces a marked toxin.

C Diff can be acquired in hospitals, or in the community, even in people not taking antibiotics. I first learned about C Diff as a fellow in infectious diseases, never imagining how often I would later encounter it in daily practice. Sometimes it's just nuisance, sometimes a life-threatening killer.

My friend Susie was on a course of antibiotics for a persistent sore throat. After two weeks, she experienced abdominal cramping and diarrhea. As soon as she stopped taking the antibiotics, her diarrhea cleared in a few days. This is a frequent pattern. In a basically healthy person, C Diff will often clear spontaneously when antibiotics are stopped.

But things were not so smooth for my patient Harry, who was in the hospital for hip surgery. He'd been prescribed antibiotics before the surgery and for a few days afterward. But when he developed explosive diarrhea, a stool sample tested positive for C Diff toxin. Harry was treated with yet another antibiotic, and his symptoms resolved. But this required four extra days in the hospital.

My chronically ill sister was diagnosed with Lyme disease and put on an intensive course of IV antibiotics. After about two weeks, she had cramping and diarrhea. After three weeks, still on IV antibiotics, she showed up at the hospital with an "acute abdomen" and was admitted to the ICU. She was going into shock, and something had to be done—immediately—to save her life. In surgery, her colon was found to be ruptured and inflamed. She barely survived and she had to live the rest of her life with a colostomy bag. Untreated C Diff was, once again, to blame.

I did not know Carol, but was asked by an attorney to be an expert witness in the lawsuit about her case. Carol, age seventy-nine, had been in the hospital following cancer surgery on the Gynecology Unit. Three nights after the operation, her blood pressure dropped and she began to experience abdominal cramping with loose stools. Overnight, this frail, elderly woman went into shock. The next morning, an "acute abdomen" of uncertain cause was diagnosed and Carol was taken to surgery. Doctors found no rupture or appendicitis, just a diffusely inflamed bowel. Surgeons closed her up, sent Carol to the ICU, and within thirty minutes an infectious disease consultant—brought in far too late—diagnosed her with C Diff colitis. Twenty-four hours later, Carol was dead. Her family filed a lawsuit.

Could any of these outcomes have been avoided? Multiple studies show that simple infection control procedures are sadly lacking in many American hospitals. The Hungarian physician Ignaz Semmelweiss[7] was the first physician to prove conclusively that hand-washing prevents hospital transmission of infection, back in the 1847. But he was ignored during his lifetime. It wasn't until the end of that century, twenty years after Semmelweiss's death, that Louis Pasteur connected bacteria to disease, inaugurating what we think of as modern medical protocols.

Yet the problems of sloppy sterilization persists. Have I been guilty myself? You bet. I wore the same white coat for more than a day and didn't routinely wipe down my stethoscope. I saw scrubs (even paper booties) being worn outside the operating room with no guarantee that they would be changed on returning to the OR.

So what's the answer? Awareness and early intervention around C Diff makes most cases fairly mild. The CDC has guidelines for preventing hospital acquired infections and the Joint Commission on Accreditation has pilot projects. But why is the infection increasing? I think poor Semmelweiss (who went insane at forty-seven, perhaps from frustration) is still wondering, "Is anyone listening to me?"

Bottom line: we *all* need reminders about washing our hands. If you feel awkward actually telling your doctor "please wash your hands," there are indirect ways to ensure this essential safety measure is followed. You can write comment cards or make phone calls to consumer relations. But I think a tactful question works best: "Say Doctor, what's your routine in the office about hand washing?"

It's not so difficult (ce n'est pas si difficile)!

DEATH IN THE RAW

I have referred throughout these pages to the importance of listening as a medical care provider of, and I mean in the fullest, which often means understanding cultures and traditions different from my own. The roots for this approach to medicine were set down early.

I remember being a medical student and spending the summer of 1962 with CARE-MEDICO's doctors and nurses in Afghanistan's Helmand valley. My focus was gathering data on infant mortality. Our jeep bumped over the dusty gravel road as we approached the small medical clinic near Lashkar Gah. Suddenly, there was a graveyard, dotted with small elongated piles of stones. Naim, our driver, noticed my confusion. "Babies, young children," was all he said.

The graveyard made real what I'd been hearing from mothers in the clinics; almost all of them had lost a child in infancy.

The sight made a deep impression on me, and it came to mind when I returned to Afghanistan three years later, in 1965, as an officer in the U.S. Public Health Service. I was assigned to the Peace Corps, eager to learn about infectious tropical diseases. Without clean water and a functional sewage system, the Afghan people were suffering fatalities from malaria, amoebic dysentery, rheumatic fever, and intestinal worms at rampant rates. About a third of patients admitted to a local hospital also had tuberculosis as a secondary diagnosis. Heart attacks were rare.

As I traveled the country caring for Peace Corps volunteers and visiting medical clinics, I also watched medical staff at work. Sometimes, it was unnerving.

In one Afghan hospital an infant arrived, sick, dehydrated, and weakly crying. He needed intravenous hydration but there were no IV fluids available. Also unavailable were sterile needles, saline, and gloves. Two Peace Corps nurses set about boiling tap water to concoct a saline IV formula. Then they boiled some used needles and 50 cc syringes. Bare handed, they placed a finger over the end of the syringe, poured in the saline, attached a needle, and injected the solution into the infant's left flank. They then repeated the procedure with the same needle, into the right flank. I was aghast at the possibility for infection. Gently, they handed the child back to his mother, who left with a sparkle of hope in her eyes, though it was likely her infant would not survive. "Tashakor," she said. (Thank you).

These experiences stayed with me. And much later in my career, after I had started a family and developed my practice in critical and pulmonary care, I jumped at the chance to return to that region of the world. In 1982, with my wife and our three grade-school aged children in tow, I accepted a position to spend my sabbatical year at the Aramco Hospital in Dhahran, Saudi Arabia.

It was a unique experience. I've alluded several times to the practice of looking for symptom patterns when attempting to identify patients' illnesses. In Saudi Arabia, I suddenly needed to learn a whole new series of them. My first three cases of what I was sure was lung cancer all turned out to be tuberculosis. Travelers returned with life threatening malaria. I saw my first case of HIV, a young man who sent us scurrying to the latest medical reports to try to treat him. But in that era, such a diagnosis was fatal. So many like him were lost.

Each day, as I drove toward the hospital for my early rounds in the ICU, I heard the morning call to prayer. Once at work, I was swept into a veritable United Nations of multiculturalism. Walking through the halls, I'd notice the lilting accents of doctors from Kerala State in India; the soft, almost demure dialect of the Filipinos; the clipped British; and English of all varieties from Egypt, Lebanon, Turkey, Sudan, and Texas. My Arabic was rudimentary so I often relied on a Palestinian translator, but sometimes I had help from Mohammed, my medical student. He was typical of the rising generation of young Shia Muslims— bright, eager to learn, but with a world view foreign to my western eyes.

As we made rounds together, Mohammed and I talked. One day, we got into a discussion about what happens after death.

"Mohammed, I view Allah as a merciful and a loving God. And the essentials of Christianity's Ten Commandments are common across religions. Don't you think that all people who try to live a good life would be welcomed into heaven?"

Mohammed met my eyes with a sympathetic look on his face.

"Jim, when you get to heaven and I'm at the right hand of Allah, I'm sorry, but you can't be admitted unless you're Muslim."

Despite our vast differences in culture, Mohammed and I respected each other and cooperated well on patient care, in which he was excelling. We walked to the bedside of one, an asthmatic woman named Sanaa (meaning "brilliance" in Arabic), who had been admitted several days prior. Her asthma attack had been severe enough to require ventilator support. But now, she'd just spent a night without sedation, in hopes that it would hasten the chances for removing her endotracheal tube and being untethered from the machine. I was surprised at her calm. Her vital signs were stable, and blood gases looked good. She seemed alert, but peaceful, and had just handwritten a series of pages.

I assumed these pieces of paper would include the usual questions and demands: "My throat is sore—when will that stop? Where am I? What happened? Let me out of here. I want my mom."

But, actually, her mom was there at the bedside, and all was calm.

I remarked on this peacefulness and asked Mohammed what Sanaa was writing.

"Jim, she has been praying, as has the family. This is not unusual. The prayers are to have Allah guide the doctors and nurses, and to help her to be content with her lot. She has been writing poetry praising Allah."

Sanaa went home with her mom three days later.

I witnessed patients like this again and again in the developing world. Many had an acceptance of disease and death that I'd rarely seen in the U.S. Perhaps it was due to lives more commonly framed by daily difficulty. Perhaps to the greater prevalence of religion in daily life.

After returning back to my practice in Seattle, I rarely had the opportunity to use most of my knowledge of tropical medicine. But once it came very much in handy. My neighbor, a Palestinian engineer named Abdul Yasu, showed up acutely ill at my E.R. early one morning when I was on call. He was wheezing, coughing, and had a high fever. His chest x-Ray showed a huge cavity, a four-inch hole, partly filled with fluid—it looked like a half-filled cup of coffee. I knew he had traveled back to his homeland, which made TB the most likely diagnosis. But this didn't look like TB. After a fair amount of sleuthing, we figured out that it was a ruptured parasitic cyst due to hydatid disease—virtually unheard of in the U.S.

My neighbor had been fortunate not to die during the rupture, which can cause an anaphylactic reaction. Now the question was, what to do?

Abdul's family insisted that I call his wife's brother, a thoracic surgeon at Hadassah Hospital in Jerusalem.

"This is absolutely common in the north, in Galilee," he said. "It must come out."

Abdul survived his surgery, and I felt grateful for that early training in parasitic diseases, which had helped me make the diagnosis. But clean water and a better sewage system in that part of the world would have prevented it altogether.

Infectious diseases continue to plague us, though they receive little attention in the media. Tuberculosis claims 1.4 million lives annually; malaria more than four hundred thousand; and HIV-AIDS nearly eight hundred thousand, the bulk of them all in low-income countries.

I suspect that while we may not know the numbers offhand, most of us sense the reality, as pointedly described on the website Our World in Data: "When it comes to the media coverage on causes of death, violent deaths account for more than two-thirds of coverage in the *New York Times* and *The Guardian* but account for less than three percent of the total deaths in the US."[8]

A BODY FOR THE MORGUE, PLEASE!

Cheryl and Susan arrived at the hospital at 6:30 AM. As was their routine, they stopped for a latte at Starbuck's and shared family stories as they walked toward the ICU. The two were well known pranksters, but widely respected as top notch nurses. The ICU, like many high-tension workplaces, can function like a family. In ours, the whole crew went to baseball games, shared picnics, and vacationed together. Cheryl and Susan were laughing as they walked into the ICU to meet up with the night shift, but they immediately sensed something amiss.

Room 3 was a disaster scene. A crash cart was there with defibrillator paddles out. All drawers had been pulled open, with multiple vials and kits removed. IV poles, procedure trays, towels, drapes, and instruments indicated a heroic but failed effort to save a patient, who was now under a sheet on a gurney.

The night crew looked devastated.

"This thirty-two-year-old woman had been admitted with severe sepsis," said Carol, the night lead, catching up Cheryl and Susan on the situation. "It was probably an abdominal abscess that ruptured. Then she bled, went in to shock, and we couldn't even get her stabilized for surgery. She died about two hours ago. Her family was a mess. So are we."

Cheryl and Susan immediately jumped into professional mode. "What can we do to help? You have a bunch of calls to make and lots of charting to do. What can we take off your plate?"

"The best thing for us now would be if you could to take the body to the morgue while we finish up here. We hate to ask but ....."

"No problem. We've got it," said Susan.

Both nurses were relieved that the family had left already, and that they were unlikely to bump into visitors. They could see the form of a fairly small woman under the sheet, but neither of them wanted to look. They were familiar with death, but this case was different. With a young woman on the gurney, it felt close to home. They were silent in the elevator as it took them down to the sub-basement where the cold lockers in the morgue were located.

The long sterile hallway leading to this area in the bowels of the hospital was dim, rubber wheels of the squeaking cart the only sound. Then they heard the noise. "Oohhhh," it moaned. They stopped and looked at each other. Gases can escape from deceased bodies, and that sometimes makes noise. But this was weird.

Another fifteen feet down the hall, the noise came again, even louder. "Oooohhhhhmmm." Then it was quiet. As they approached the morgue doors, it came again, "ooooohhhmmm," and the body began to sit up!

Cheryl and Susan had had enough. Screaming, they both ran, leaving the body now upright on the cart. They tore down the hall, straight into the arms of their colleagues, who were breaking up with laughter. The "body," a colleague, climbed off the cart running after them with glee.

Gallows humor is endemic to many high-stress occupations. Fire stations, police precincts, and news rooms are famous for it. If we can laugh, it seems, we can work through conditions that might feel daunting otherwise. I often think of George Bernard Shaw, who observed: "Life does not cease to be funny when people die, any more than it ceases to be serious when people laugh."[9]

THE TB BLUES

After my fellowship in infectious diseases, I decided to learn more about tuberculosis (TB) and took a position running the admitting ward at the local TB sanatorium in Seattle—a teaching hospital for medical students and medical residents. Our patients were a mix of foreign-born ex-pats, alcoholics, homeless, and Native Americans. TB is classically a disease of poverty and continues to be one of the top killers in the world, taking more than one million lives per year. During the 1970s, as TB began to be controlled in the U.S., hospitals dedicated to its treatment closed. Most people believed TB would be eliminated in this country by 2025.

The cases I saw often presented in atypical ways. Sometimes, a patient would have TB that had laid dormant for decades, since childhood, but became activated when their immune system was stressed—for whatever reason. I saw exactly this in a Philippine-born bank executive who came to me with a fever, voice change, and cough. But his chest x-ray was suspicious for TB. Upon examination, I was startled to see a bulging mass in the back of his throat. It pushed his tongue forward and narrowed the airway. A second x-ray and CT scan showed that the infection had invaded the vertebrae of his neck. It turned out that my patient had TB of the cervical spine as well as pulmonary TB. He responded beautifully to modern TB drugs, but treatment is typically months long. He followed the regimen faithfully for half a year and was cured.

A seventeen-year-old girl was brought in on a stretcher in 1971, with wasting, fatigue, pallor, cough, and a diffusely abnormal x-ray. She had been seen at her home by her MD uncle, who thought she had pneumonia. By the time I met her, the TB was far advanced, and this teenager was near death. Standard drugs, vitamins, good food, and bed rest resulted, eventually, in a recovery. But my patient spent two years in treatment and permanently lost 60% of her lung function. It is essential that TB be caught early.

TB is the great masquerader and can show up literally anywhere, not just the lungs. A seventy-year-old woman from India developed fever, confusion, and neck stiffness before falling into coma. A spinal tap was suspicious for TB, but not proven. Aggressive treatment for TB allowed her to recover and return home. Similarly, a diabetic patient presented the hospital with severe lower abdominal pain. Exploratory surgical of her abdomen was unrevealing, but when we reviewed her abdominal x-rays, we found that two of her spinal vertebrae showed destruction from TB. Her abdominal pain was due to nerves from the vertebrae sending pain signals to the lower abdomen.

Her treatment and cure were straightforward. But I had another patient who awoke at night, spewing blood from his mouth. He'd been in the hospital for a large TB cavity in his lung, and now a large artery near the cavity had ruptured. This man died within minutes, despite our vigorous efforts to save him—a sad example of what should only be in the medical history books.

Should we all have the "TB Blues"?[10] If you listen to this 1931 classic by Jimmie Rodgers, who died from the disease, I think you'd agree that we should. Tuberculosis existed in ancient Egypt and may even be referenced in the Bible: "The Lord will smite you with consumption and with fever, inflammation, and fiery heat...." Many well-known authors, artists, and musicians have suffered its ravages. Perhaps the most notable family is the Brontes, including Maria Bronte, (mother of the famed writers) who died at age thirty-eight; her daughter, also Maria, who died at eleven; another daughter, Elizabeth, died at twelve; Bramwell died at thirty; Emily (author of *Wuthering Heights*), at twenty-nine; Anne at twenty-seven; and Charlotte (who wrote *Jane Eyre*) died of tuberculosis and complications in pregnancy at thirty-nine.

Yet TB remains a modern plague in much of the world, particularly where there is poverty or social disruption. Crowded housing and lack of robust public health systems allow TB to spread unchecked. Despite its roots in ancient history, even today 10 million become ill with TB each year. The latest alarming wrinkle is that the bug has developed resistance to multiple drugs.

No one had a clue about the cause of tuberculosis until the little-known German physician Robert Koch astounded the scientific world with proof that the TB bacillus was a distinct organism that could be transmitted from animal to animal (guinea pigs). Prior to his discovery, TB was not considered an infectious disease at all. No one even realized that the TB bacillus existed. Koch won the Nobel Prize[11] in Medicine for his discovery, in 1905.

So what's being done? The Bill & Melinda Gates Foundation has been attacking the disease for years. Many medical schools are focusing renewed attention on TB. And organizations like the Center for Infectious Disease Research Institute are working toward its prevention (through vaccines), novel identification, and targeted drug management. Paul Farmer's book, *Mountains*

Beyond Mountains, discusses his personal attempts to battle TB in Haiti, outlining new hope for workable programs.

But the fact is that the idea of eliminating tuberculosis in the U.S. by 2025 was overly optimistic. Attempts to control it continue to thwart medicine because TB continues to be associated with poverty, poor housing, and lack of access to medical care. It is as much as a sociopolitical problem as it is a medical conundrum.

A VISITOR IN THE OPERATING ROOM

Strange things happen in hospitals that we never hear about. It's not all about death and dying. Some stories never get told—but I can't forget this one. I was chief of specialty services when the director of nursing said to me, "You've got to do something about this!"

It was Trevor's first weekend to relax since moving to Seattle. He was out in a park, walking Bailey, his year-old lab, when his pager beeped. Trevor called in to the operating room office, where the frantic head nurse told him he needed to come in. The scheduled anesthesiologist was ill with the flu, and no one else could cover. Trevor would need to come in for at least two cases, perhaps more.

"Can you find anyone else?" he asked. "It's my first weekend off, and I doubt that I'll be able to find anyone to watch Bailey."

"Sorry, we need you—now," came the curt reply.

Trevor hadn't gotten to know his neighbors yet, so he could hardly ask them to take care of Bailey. Having no other choice, he packed the dog, along with water and food, into his Subaru, hoping that the pooch wouldn't mind hanging out in the car for a while.

Trevor parked the car in the shade, cracked the windows, and headed for the OR, with Bailey barking from the car. The case lasted only an hour, and Trevor quickly headed back out to his car. Bailey was tearing it up. There were scratch marks on the door and a tear in the seat cover. This just wasn't going to work.

So Trevor walked Bailey around to the back of the hospital, entered the service entrance, and took the back service elevator, which came up just outside the anesthesia call room. He stayed with Bailey, making sure that he had water, food and a comfortable pillow to lie on. Then it was off to the next case. Bailey seemed content to wait.

The case was an appendectomy. The patient was anesthetized in the usual fashion, and Trevor settled in to watch the monitors while the surgeon went to work. Strangely, he felt a sudden pressure and a cold wet sensation on his left leg. Looking down, he found Bailey, looking up at his master, tail wagging with joy.

"Where in the hell did that dog come from?" screeched the OR nurse. "Get him out of here!"

The surgeon didn't miss a beat. "At least give him a mask and dog booties."

Trevor's anesthetized patient, of course, was peacefully oblivious.

Security officers took over babysitting for Bailey until Trevor could leave, red faced. I'm happy to report that the unsuspecting patient did well, Trevor kept his job, and Bailey probably wondered what the fuss was all about.

IT WAS RIGHT IN PLAIN SIGHT

Jacob, a family practitioner colleague, had been admitted to our Coronary Care Unit with a heart attack. Fortunately, he was improving day by day. But one of the nurses, concerned, called me in to watch his breathing. She wasn't sure what was going on. Jacob would snore, stop breathing, snort, and start inhaling again. Correspondingly, his oxygen levels cycled up and then down to alarmingly low levels. This happened at least once every minute.

This was back in 1981, and in our departmental meeting, we had just reviewed the first publication about CPAP in the *Lancet*, written by the inventor of the process, Dr. Collin Sullivan. He described sleep apnea and its treatment with positive air pressure—an amazingly simple yet brilliant solution. CPAP design had not advanced to the point of comfort for the patient, so we had to cobble together fairly primitive equipment to treat Jacob.

But we were amazed to see his snoring resolve and the oxygen levels normalize. He felt more rested than he had for years.

It's not often than we have a new disease discovered, let alone a treatment without dangerous side effects. And it had been hiding in plain sight! Subsequent research confirmed what we suspected—a lot of people have sleep apnea, approximately three percent to seven percent of adult men and two percent to five percent of adult women.

By the 1990s our department, which added the specialty of sleep medicine, was inundated with requests for sleep apnea evaluation. In response, we developed a procedure for home testing, which I was able to discuss with the Stanford physician William Dement, known as the father of sleep medicine. He supported the concept. Home testing has since become commonplace, though overnight sleep evaluations in a laboratory are still necessary for more complex sleep disorders.

I have frequently been asked, "Can sleep apnea kill you?" The short answer is yes. People with severe sleep apnea have a much higher mortality risk than those without the condition. Risk of death increases when sleep apnea is untreated. In a large population study, about 42% of deaths in people with severe sleep apnea were attributed to cardiovascular disease or stroke (compared with rates of 26% for people with no sleep apnea). Obesity is a common underlying factor.[12]

Another patient, Joe, was referred to my clinic urgently. He was a fork lift operator. The previous day at work, he'd had a large load high in the air, but then all went quiet. He awoke to yelling in his headphones: "Dammit Joe, wake up before you kill someone!"

Joe wasn't unusual. Truck drivers have warned me to steer clear of big rigs on the highway. "We do nod off from time to time," one admitted.

Joe's home study revealed severe sleep apnea. His airway would close off sixty times an hour, and each time his oxygen saturation dipped toward 60%. (Normal is well above 90%.) Joe was placed on a self-adjusting CPAP system. Delighted with his results, he

confessed that his wife could finally sleep through the night without continually poking him or having to move to the couch.

Discovering a new, non-infectious and easily treatable disease
is almost unheard of in the modern era, and we are now finding
additional uses for CPAP technology. In hospitalized patients with
severe COVID-19 pneumonia, CPAP has been used in place of
the much more invasive ventilator. The same technology has also
been modified and upgraded to a bi-level device (BiPAP) to provide non-invasive ventilation for a variety of respiratory disorders.
The keen observations of Dr. Sullivan have improved millions of
lives, and prevented many deaths.

EXCESSIVE USE OF "HEALTH CARE"

Ask almost any doctor or nurse, and they can tell stories about
mess-ups in health care. Sometimes, it's underutilization, sometimes the wrong treatment or test is done, and sometimes it's inap-
propriate overuse of tests or treatments.

I was discussing this with an ophthalmologist recently. He had
been working for a large medical group. One day an administrator
met with them telling them that he was concerned about high
overhead costs and the "inadequate" revenue being generated. The
eleven ophthalmologists were told directly that they weren't billing enough and thus they weren't meeting their targets. The doctors pointed out that they were providing excellent high-quality
care for their patients.

"Listen, you folks just don't get it," the administrator snapped.
"If you have a patient in the office and there's a billable procedure,
DO IT!"

Six of the doctors rebelled and left the group, after announcing
that they wanted to practice within both legal and ethical boundaries—impossible, they said, in a procedure-driven environment.

When I was scouting around for my first job in internal medicine, a group of doctors asked me if I was interested in becoming
their "thyroid guy." They had just purchased a thyroid scanner

and felt they had a golden opportunity to generate a revenue stream from Medicare and insurance billing. I wondered if they'd gone into medicine with these kinds of aims, or if they'd once had more idealism about the field. If so, when had they abandoned it?

"The estimated cost of waste in the U.S. health care system ranges from $760 billion to $935 billion, accounting for approximately 25% of total health care spending," according to a 2019 study published in JAMA.[13] How do we begin to change this behavior? All of us have ideas—among them, revising incentives, tort reform, more evidence-based research, primary care teams and guidelines for use of expert opinions. None of the current proposals for reform effectively deal with overuse of scarce and costly resources. Our whole system is built on a profit motive—more visits, more tests, and more procedures all lead to more income.

Having my own health coverage under Medicare now, I do appreciate this version of socialized medicine. It is too costly at present, but provides a framework that will work if we can successfully address overuse and price gouging. Double-digit cost increases for health care every year are simply not sustainable; like it or not, an end will come. Let's hope the public discourse can be rational. Most doctors just want to practice good medicine, with good colleagues, in a good system.

LEAVING A LEGACY

*P*art of dying is hoping that we are leaving something positive behind. Have we taken the time to do this? My mom set an example for those she loved.

A LETTER FOR MY LOVED ONES

Death at age eighty-four can be peaceful and expected, or sudden and tragic. My mom's was the latter. She had been in the ICU after having an abdominal aortic aneurysm repaired, a major operation for someone in this age group (nowadays many of these are handled by less invasive techniques). I flew to Philadelphia and was with her for the first four days after the operation. She was frail, but stable, when I returned to Seattle.

The next day, my dad received a call from the hospital. Mom had suffered a cardiac arrest and CPR was ineffective.

When all of this was relayed to me, I reeled with emotions: sadness that I wasn't there with her; worry that she'd suffered; grief for my dad. And behind it all, the nagging question of whether her surgeon had been competent.

I flew back to Pennsylvania for the funeral. The memorial service was held in the beautiful Bryn Athyn Cathedral. The Swedenborgian service was upbeat, though it didn't deny our sense of loss.

Someone said to me, "We Swedenborgians are among those who cry tears of joy at weddings and laugh though our sadness at funerals as we picture our loved one awakening in the next life."

The burial was a simple affair. A nephew offered to hand carve the headstone. The burial site, in the old Bryn Athyn graveyard near Pennypack Creek where deer roamed, looked more like a path through the woods.

Dad, at eighty-seven, was in a daze. He looked lost, and we needed to make plans rapidly for extra care. The hardest thing was going through all of mom's old papers. We knew she had typed up a family history, sketched out genealogy trees, and collected volumes of papers from all us kids, including report cards all the way back to first grade.

Then we found the letter. It was in a sealed envelope with no stamp. "In case anything happens to me" was written across the front. My siblings and I were stunned. It took a while to gather everyone together and read it. But what an experience Mom left us. She had written a love letter to Dad, with affectionate references to all of us and our spouses. We could hear her talking, urging us to love one another, not to chase after worldly possessions, and to lead useful lives. She even chastised herself for always nagging us to do more. There were no hints of accusation or regret—only love. We had discovered our legacy.

A VALUE STATEMENT IN YOUR ADVANCE DIRECTIVE

One day in my office, an elderly couple presented me with a document that they wanted to add to their advance directives:

"I have a firm belief that God created me, that there is a natural cycle of life, that death is inevitable, and that dying should be peaceful, comfortable, at home, if possible, and without tubes, artificial nutrition or ventilator support. If I cannot carry out self-care, do not have my usual mental faculties, have an incurable disease or intractable pain, please treat me with the best care for comfort but not invasive life support. It is quite acceptable to withhold fluid and nutrition from me and treat me with a morphine drip as part of this care for comfort, letting nature take its course. I have no wish to be a burden to my loved ones, or to spend resources and energy on heroic efforts to prolong my life when life is at end. Only in the acute situation (e.g. trauma) would I want aggressive care. It would be a nightmare to spend my days in a nursing home with a feeding tube. Quality, not quantity, of earthly life is more important."

I was impressed that they'd taken the initiative to start this conversation with me. Their statement was clear and commanding. It said: please listen and pay attention!

You can add something like this to your Living Will at any time. It will be a useful guide for your physician and loved ones. It also promotes conversations focused on values, not only on whatever high-tech, marginally beneficial treatment *could* be attempted. Such a document can help inform bedside decisions which can be difficult and nuanced.

THE ETHICAL WILL

Have you ever thought about what you want to leave behind? I'm not referring to estate planning exactly. I'm talking about a legacy that is uniquely yours that you'd like others to know about. Perhaps you can be an influence on another life as yours is ending.

An Ethical Will is a powerful way to leave a positive legacy of your thoughts and values. I encouraged patients to consider writing one while doing end-of-life planning, so that more of us might receive a love letter from beyond like the one my mom left. Hospice physician Dr. Barry Baines[14] has been a leader in this endeavor promoting Ethical Wills as a way "to pass on one's legacy of wisdom and legacy of generosity, as well as the legacy of values..."

In the past, oral tradition played that role, then it was written letters. Now it's digital media.

A non-profit called StoryCorps[15] is leading a nationwide effort to bridge the generational divide by providing the opportunity to record, share, and preserve stories of our lives. When we leave these narratives behind, our voices live on. I think this work has provided us something like a national Ethical Will—a mix of stories with values embedded to pass on to future generations.

One day a few years back, the StoryCorps airstream trailer with its portable recording studio drove up to the Bill & Melinda Gates Foundation. My daughter, who worked there, had arranged to interview my wife about growing up abroad and coming to the U.S. for her education—capturing part of the immigrant experience. This was a gift to our family and hopefully it will be to others in the future.

The Ethical Will can be a spiritual or moral legacy. It can also be incorporated into advance directives for end-of-life decision making, helping the doctor at your bedside to know you. The more modern way is to video a loved one talking through thoughts about the issues that made them who they are—similar to the experience of my wife and daughter with StoryCorps. Not to be outdone, one of my sons recently set up his video camera in our living room saying, "Mom and Dad, it's time to talk. I want to know your story."

AFTERWORD:
GRIEF AND RESILIENCE

What about the future of death? Pandemics notwithstanding, it will soon become common to live to one hundred—a silver tsunami that society is not prepared for. Burial and cremation will become rarer as access to human composting[1] gains traction as a "green" solution. The more we learn about the cellular mechanisms of aging, the more people will attempt to find ways of staving them off to live indefinitely—with unintended consequences we cannot now imagine. And I am confident that medical aid in dying will become mainstream across the country as we recognize that the right to die is like any other right we hold dear. At the same time, hospice and palliative care will expand, providing services to all who need them.

That's the good news. But before we get there, the crisis of long-term care for the aged will worsen, eating up more of our life savings. The health aspects of climate change, meanwhile, will become severe. While some of us will glimpse the future of technology and its effects on longevity, the scourges of worldwide poverty, malnutrition, war, and infectious diseases will continue to decimate millions of others who live "out of sight, out of mind" in the developing world. We were poorly prepared for the COVID-19 pandemic, and I see no reason to think we will be any better positioned for the next natural disaster.

But as individuals, we are always learning. Recently, two elderly friends told me how they dealt with loss.

One of them was Rita. Her husband, John, had been in a memory care unit for five years. Rita buzzed around with her walker after spinal surgery, worked vigorously with physical therapy, and now was regularly attending the symphony. Every evening she spent with John, watching TV or listening to music. He no longer knew who she was or where they were, but she could laugh and tell me stories about their encounters. Often, he would look at her quizzically and ask, "Are we married?"

"Yes."

"Well, that's nice!"

One Friday evening, John became ill, and Rita took him to the nearest hospital, which happened to be Harborview Medical Center, a level-one trauma care facility. Harborview's E.R. is famously hectic. John and Rita were surrounded by incoming patients with knife and gunshot wounds, the mentally ill, and many unfortunate people unable to get routine medical care any other way.

When they returned to their room at the memory care facility John remarked, "Boy that was some party we went to!"

"Sure was."

"But, you know, I don't think we should invite those people over to our place," John concluded.

Rita cackled as she told this story. She loved John. She wasn't making fun of him. She was simply able to put humor into the pathos of their situation. We all have adaptive capabilities, and in adversity they are often strengthened.

Then there's ninety-year-old Alice, whom I ran into at a memorial. "I've lost two husbands and three sons, and somehow I'm still going," she said.

I was incredulous. "How do you do it?"

"Well, I've always been a glass-half-full person, and always enjoyed having fun. I spent my life as a teacher. The kids kept me young. In fact, I can tell you a story you might not believe."

"Go on, please."

"I was a high school substitute for an English class and had to step out in the hall for a message one day. When I returned to the classroom someone had written F-U-C-K on the black-board. Some of the kids were smiling. Some looked afraid. Others seemed angry. I said, 'do you know what FUCK stands for?' You could have heard a pin drop. 'It's an acronym,' I told them: For Unlawful Carnal Knowledge. Then I moved straight into a discussion of Stegner."

"Wow. Was there any blowback?"

"After class, I told the principal, who laughed. He said, 'Let's just see what happens.'"

"And?"

"Not a word from anyone. Years later, I ran into one of those students and asked if she remembered the 'F-incident.' 'Oh, yes!' she said. I asked why no parents had complained and she told me, 'Are you kidding? None of us would ever have told that story to our parents!'"

Alice considered experiences like this the key to hanging on to a youthful outlook. I'd call them lessons in resilience and flexibility. But she was not done teaching me.

"Don't talk about closure," Alice said, referring to the ways we typically struggle to handle death, "And don't make gratuitous comments like 'I'm sure they're in a better place.'"

"Ok, Alice. But I still don't really get how you have weathered so much loss and kept going," I said, feeling a bit thick.

"Actually, it's all about Brussels sprouts. I hate them, and my late husband loved them. I'm just so happy to wake up every day knowing that I don't have to cook them anymore," she said with a chuckle.

We naturally search for resilience during experiences of grief and loss. Moving forward when our feet are heavy can seem like a hurdle too high. Friendship, humor, exercise, and volunteering all help. But the best medicine is love—the warmth of close human connections. Alice found a way to keep going forward through a mix of all these ingredients—and her appreciation of being free from Brussels sprouts.

APPENDIX -
FAQS

There are numerous books, websites, pamphlets, and videos about advance care planning. I have listed a few that I find most useful in guiding people through thinking about the following questions:

How can I have a conversation about death and dying with my loved ones?

The Conversation Project was started by Pulitzer Prize-winning author Ellyn Goodman. It could be your "one stop shop" for advance care planning. www.theconversationproject.org.

Advance care directives look complicated. Do I have to have one?

No, you don't have to have one, but you should! I hope after reading this book that you will.

What's the most important thing to do in preparing for death?

More important than completing any document is designating your advocate. First, have a heart-to-heart conversation with the person you'd like to be your Durable Power of Attorney for Health Care. Talk it through and ask if they are willing to serve in this capacity. Then sign, have witnesses, and notarize the document in accordance with the requirements of your state. Your advocate will speak for you when you cannot speak for yourself. This is who I, as an attending physician, would turn to at the bedside for guidance if you cannot provide it.

Where can I find the forms?

I have found Prepare for Your Care the most useful site. It has many helpful vid-eos about your choices. This site has advance directive forms in English and Spanish for every state. The forms can be down-loaded and printed or filled out and stored on line. This site provides a method for combining the value statement, a living will, and your durable power of attorney into a single docu-ment valid in your state. www.prepareforyourcare.org.

Are there specific directives for dementia?

The Advance Directive for Dementia is the least complicated one to complete and is proving to be popular and useful. https://dementia-directive.org/.

Can I get help filling out the documents?

You can make an appointment with your medical provider to discuss and clarify your wishes about end-of-life care. Many hospitals and clinics also offer classes. Organizations like Honoring Choices (https://www.honoringchoicespnw.org/) and Respecting Choices (https://respectingchoices.org/) focus on education.

Should I complete a POLST/MOLST form?

If you have a serious illness, are very frail or feel that you don't have long to live, this form can express your wishes. It's most useful in telling emergency responders what you would or wouldn't want in terms of life support. It needs to be signed by you and your medical provider. This document then becomes legal standing orders for your medical care. https://polst.org/.

I'm DNR status and want no CPR or ventilator. Will that be honored?

First make sure you complete the POLST/MOLST form described above. Then make sure your advocate and health care provider have copies of the form. Display your own copy in a prominent place. Consider buying a DNR bracelet or medallion that will clearly display your DNR status when the POLST/MOLST is not immediately available.

What should I do with these documents?

Copies of your advance directives should be available in your home, your doctor's office, and with your advocate. It's useful to discuss them with all members of your family. These documents should be updated every decade, at least, and certainly if your health is worsening, or in the event of a serious life event. Ask your doctor's office to store them as part of your electronic medical record, and ask how they can be accessed 24/7 in case of an emergency.

How do doctors make decisions in the ICU? Will they listen?

A social worker and I published a Patient Care Conference Guide about shared decision-making in the ICU. Doctors work with you or your advocate to follow your wishes. This is when your advocate is so important. Ethically, doctors need to listen. But have you told them all they need to know?
http://digitalcommons.hamline.edu/hlr/vol36/iss2/13/.

Are there legal concerns in end-of-life decision making?

Law Professor Thaddeus Pope, in his legal blog, offers commentary on the evolving legal issues around end-of-life care. There are also elder law attorneys who specialize in this area. http://medicalfutility.blogspot.com/.

What other plans should I make?

Depending on how detailed you want to be, it may be helpful to think about what you want for funeral arrangements and a memorial service. Some people choose the venue, music, readings, and food ahead of time. Others leave it up to their loved ones.

Where can I read more?

Being Mortal by Dr. Atul Gawande has long been my favorite book. Gawande writes about the issues of death and dying in a warm, humanistic way.

Dying Well by Dr. Ira Byock offers practical advice from a hospice physician.

Many other books are listed at https://theconversationproject. org/tcp-blog/10-must-reads-about-death-and-end-of-life-care/

My blog has many stories from my years in practice, some of which are now in this book. www.endoflifeblog.com

Are there helpful videos or movies about death and dying?

The movies *Endgame* (Netflix) and *Dying at Grace* are both worthwhile.

The video *Extremis* (Netflix) follows Dr. Jessica Nutik Vitter, who is both a critical care and palliative care physician, discussing death with patients.

I appear briefly in a documentary film, which follows several patients on their journey toward death. https://speakingofdying.com /speaking-of-dying-film-dying-well/

How do I contact hospice?

If you even think you might benefit from hospice services, ask your doctor to refer you, or call a local hospice yourself to get more information. Follow the dictum: think hospice, and think about it early. https://hospicefoundation.org/Hospice-Care/Hospice-Services.

How do I contact palliative care?

Your physician can refer you to a palliative care specialist. Please ask to see one if your pain or other symptoms are not well controlled.

Where can I get information about MAID or VSED?

The national organization, Compassion and Choices, advocates for end-of-life choices. Its staff and volunteers can direct you to local resources and physicians, help you to understand your options, and provide support for your decisions. https://compassionandchoices.org/.

I have a family member in a nursing home. How do I find an Ombudsman?

Every state has protections for residents of nursing homes. Don't hesitate to ask to see the Ombudsman in your area if concerns aren't being addressed satisfactorily. https://theconsumervoice .org/get_help.

How does organ donation work? Can I be a donor?

https://www.organdonor.gov/about/process.html

I'd like to attend an event to discuss end-of-life issues with others. Is that possible?

Let's Have Dinner and Talk About Death: This group offers popular, somewhat scripted dinners with several others, usually in a private home. http://www.deathoverdinner.org/

Death Café: This is a meet-up group that gathers in public cafés for discussions similar to the dinner table talks described above, but in a less formal setting. www.deathcafe.com.

The End Well Project shares innovative ideas to inspire new thinking about the end of life. https://endwellproject.org/

NOTES

INTRODUCTION

1 Krakauer E, Penson RT, Truog RD, et al. Sedation for intractable distress of a dying patient: acute palliative care and the principle of double effect. Oncologist. 2000; 5:53–62.

2 An Official American Thoracic Society Clinical Policy Statement: Palliative Care for Patients with Respiratory Diseases and Critical Illnesses. AJRCCM. 2008; 8:912-927.

3 13Vacco v Quill, 117 S. Ct 2293(1997).

4 Beauchamp TL, The Right to Die as the Triumph of Autonomy. J Med Philos. 2006; 31(6):643-654

5 https://www.theonion.com/world-death-rate-holding-steady-at-100-percent -1819564171

6 Sherwin B. Nuland, *How We Die: Reflections on Life's Final Chapter* (Random House, Inc.; New York, 1994)

A TIME TO DIE

1 https://digitalcommons.hamline.edu/hlr/vol36/iss2/13/

2 http://medicalfutility.blogspot.com/

3 Smith AK, Lo B. The Problem with Actually Tattooing DNR across Your Chest. J Gen Intern Med 2012;27:1238–1239

4 Yaguchi A, Truog R, Curtis JR. International Differences in End-of-Life Attitudes in the Intensive Care Unit. Arch Intern Med 2005;165:1970-1975

5 Curtis JR , Kross EK, Stapleton RD. The Importance of Addressing Advance Care Planning and Decisions About Do-Not-Resuscitate Orders During Novel Coronavirus 2019 (COVID-19). JAMA 2020;10:1001

6 Jameton A. What Moral Distress in Nursing History Could Suggest About the Future of Health Care; AMA J of Ethics 2017;6:617-628.

7 Rushton CH. AACN Adv Crit Care 2016;27 (1):111–119.

8 https://www.nejm.org/doi/full/10.1056/NEJMc1911892

9 https://www.waombudsman.org/residents-rights/

LEARNING TO LISTEN

1 https://deathcafe.com

2 https://deathoverdinner.org

3 https://prepareforyourcare.org/welcome

4 Zier LS, Sottile PD, Hong SY, et al. Surrogate Decision Makers' Interpretation of Prognostic Information: A Mixed-Methods Study. Ann Intern Med 2012;156(5):360-366

5 First published in the Journal of the American Medical Association (JAMA); Published in Giraffe under a Grey Sky, 2010, Rockingham Press

CONFLICTS

1 Guidelines for the determination of death: Report of the medical consultants on the diagnosis of death to the President's commission for the study of ethical problems in medicine and biomedical and behavioral research. JAMA 1981;246:2184–6

2 https://www.npr.org/sections/health-shots/2016/12/26/499494248/a -dying-man-s-wish-to-donate-his-organs-gets-complicated

3 Tilburt JC, Emanuel EJ, Kaptchuk TJ, et al. Prescribing 'placebo treatments': results of a national survey of US internists and rheumatologists. BMJ 2008;337:a1938

4 https://www.newyorker.com/magazine/2011/12/12/the-power-of -nothing

5 https://www.mcgill.ca/oss/article/controversial-science-health-history -news/would-osler-stand-his-famous-quote-today

6 https://dementia-directive.org/

7 https://www.pbs.org/newshour/show/unequal-medical-treatment

8 Doug Wojcieszak, James W Saxton, Esq., Maggie M Finkelstein, *Sorry Works*. (AuthorHouse 2008)

9 Wu AW, Cavanaugh TA, McPhee S J, et al. To tell the truth. J GEN INTERN MED 1997;12:770–775 https://www.ncbi.nlm.nih.gov/pmc/articles /PMC1497204/pdf/jgi_7163.pdf

ASSISTANCE IN DYING—PROS AND CONS

1 Ira Byock, *Dying Well, Peace and Possibilities at the End of Life;* (Riverhead Books, New York, 1997)

2 Jessica Nutik Zitter, *Extreme Measures, finding a better path to the end of life*; (Penguin Random House, New York, 2017)

3 http://w2.vatican.va/content/john-paul-ii/en/encyclicals/documents/hf_jp-ii_enc_25031995_evangelium-vitae.html

4 https://www.canada.ca/en/health-canada/services/medical-assistance-dying.html

5 https://www.washingtontimes.com/news/2017/jun/14/obamacare-death-panels-should-be-ended/

6 https://www.ascopost.com/issues/june-25-2018/voluntarily-stopping-eating-and-drinking-is-legal-and-ethical/

7 https://www.ncbi.nlm.nih.gov/pmc/articles/PMC5916258/

8 https://www.cdc.gov/nchs/fastats/leading-causes-of-death.htm

9 https://khn.org/news/suicide-seniors-long-term-care-nursing-homes/

10 https://khn.org/news/rational-suicide-seniors-preemptive-death-medical-aid-in-dying/

11 https://www.ncbi.nlm.nih.gov/pmc/articles/PMC2685270/

12 http://www.bioethics.net/2019/05/a-tribute-for-dax-cowart-1947-2019/

13 Curtis RJ, Burt RA. Chest 2007; 132(3):748-751; discussion 755-756

14 Peabody FW. JAMA 1927;88(12):877-882.

15 https://www.theatlantic.com/magazine/archive/2014/10/why-i-hope-to-die-at-75/379329/

REFLECTIONS

1 http://www.theisticscience.org/spirituality/Ingersoll3.htm

2 Helen Keller, *Light In My Darkness*, (Swedenborg Foundation, 2000)

3 Mark Twain, *Notebooks and Journals*, vol. 3

4 Mark Twain, *Captain Stormfield's Visit to Heaven*, (Harper and Brothers, 1907}

5 McNeil, Jr. What the Next Year (or Two) May Look Like. New York Times; April 19, 2020

6 Gorbach SL, Bartlett JG. Contributions to the Discovery of Clostridium difficile Antibiotic-Associated Diarrhea. Clin Infect Dis 2014;59:S66–S70.

7 https://www.britannica.com/biography/Ignaz-Semmelweis

8 https://ourworldindata.org/causes-of-death#does-the-news-reflect-what-we-die-from

9 Bernard Shaw, *The Doctor's Dilemma*, (Penguin 1946).

10 https://www.youtube.com/watch?v=UcVOYPUL5S4

11 https://www.nobelprize.org/prizes/medicine/1905/koch/biographical/

12 https://aasm.org/study-shows-that-people-with-sleep-apnea-have-a-high-risk-of-death/

13 Shrank WH, Rogstad TL, Parekh N. JAMA. 2019;322(15):1501-1509.
14 Barry K Baines, *Ethical Wills*, (Da Capo Press, 2006)
15 https://storycorps.org/participate/

AFTERWORD: GRIEF AND RESILIENCE

1 https://www.smithsonianmag.com/smart-news/washington-first-state
-allow-burial-method-human-composting-180972020/

ACKNOWLEDGMENTS

My heartfelt thanks to those who reviewed and supported this book: Shannon Lorah, Jeannie Fessenden RN, Rev. Elizabeth Graham, Dr. Ann Milam, Sharmon Figgenshaw ARNP and Mary Catlin. Group Health Cooperative (now Kaiser Permanente) has supported me with ethics training and in the development of an educational program for patients called "Your Life Your Choices." Monique Shira helped me understand the language of social media. I learned the skill of talking to patients about their end of life choices in working with Joi Murotani Dennett, the co-chair of our hospital ethics committee.

Greg Shaw, my friend, writer, and publisher, has encouraged and supported me from the first idea for this book and continues to support me through his team at Clyde Hill Publishing. My editor, Claudia Rowe, has helped in countless ways to provide the "connective tissue" linking my stories and clarifying their message. Dr. Eric Larson, who wrote the forward, gave me new insights on the meaning of death. Thanks also to the many outstanding people I've been molded by: professors, colleagues, nurses, social workers, and respiratory therapists. The outstanding Department of Pulmonary, Critical Care and Sleep Medicine at the University of Washington has supported my interest in teaching over the years keeping me on as a Clinical Professor, Emeritus even as I've aged into an old man. My greatest teachers, though, were my patients. Over time they told me stories, broadened my horizons and taught me how to care for them. Lastly, my wife, Lourdes, has graciously supported my efforts and has helped me to redefine my life's goals: "Don't worry about success—just be kind."

ABOUT THE AUTHOR

Dr. Jim deMaine practiced pulmonary and critical care medicine in the Seattle area for more than three decades. After graduating from the University of Pennsylvania School of Medicine, he served as a commissioned officer in the United States Public Health Service, spending two years assigned to the Peace Corps in Afghanistan. Dr. deMaine spent much of his career as chief of medical specialties and co-chair of the ethics committee at Group Health Cooperative (now Kaiser Permanente). He is a Professor of Medicine Emeritus at the University of Washington School of Medicine where he has worked with medical students and physicians in training. He lives with his wife in Seattle. They have three adult children and six grandchildren.

9 781734 979107